Spine Surgery Vivas for the FRCS (TR & Orth)

Spine Surgery Vivas for the FRCS (Tr & Orth)

Kelechi Eseonu
BSc (Hons), MSc (Oxon), FRCS (Tr and Orth)
Senior Clinical Fellow in Spinal Surgery, St Michael's Hospital, Canada

Nicolas Beresford-Cleary
MBChB, BEng, FRCS (Tr and Orth)
Senior Clinical Fellow in Spinal Surgery, Vancouver General Hospital, Canada

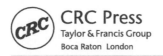
CRC Press
Taylor & Francis Group
Boca Raton London

CRC Press is an imprint of the
Taylor & Francis Group, an **informa** business

First edition published 2022
by CRC Press
6000 Broken Sound Parkway NW, Suite 300, Boca Raton, FL 33487–2742

and by CRC Press
2 Park Square, Milton Park, Abingdon, Oxon, OX14 4RN

© 2022 Taylor & Francis Group, LLC

CRC Press is an imprint of Taylor & Francis Group, LLC

Library of Congress Cataloging-in-Publication Data
Names: Eseonu, Kelechi, author. | Beresford-Cleary, Nicolas, author.
Title: Spine surgery Vivas for the FRCS (Tr & Orth) / Kelechi Eseonu, Nicolas Beresford-Cleary.
Description: First edition | Boca Raton : CRC Press, 2022. | Includes bibliographical references and index.
Identifiers: LCCN 2021032672 (print) | LCCN 2021032673 (ebook) | ISBN 9781032062310 (paperback) |
    ISBN 9781032062358 (hardback) | ISBN 9781003201304 (ebook)
Subjects: MESH: Spine—surgery | Spinal Diseases—surgery | Examination Questions | Case Reports
Classification: LCC RD533 (print) | LCC RD533 (ebook) | NLM WE 18.2 | DDC 617.4/71—dc23
LC record available at https://lccn.loc.gov/2021032672
LC ebook record available at https://lccn.loc.gov/2021032673

ISBN: 978-1-032-06235-8 (hbk)
ISBN: 978-1-032-06231-0 (pbk)
ISBN: 978-1-003-20130-4 (ebk)

DOI: 10.1201/9781003201304

Typeset in Minion Pro
by Apex CoVantage, LLC

CONTENTS

PREFACE

Written by two fellowship-trained spinal surgeons who have recently passed the FRCS (Tr and Orth), this book aims to prepare candidates for the spinal vivas in the exam. Whilst spine surgery may be less familiar to many trainees than trauma or arthroplasty, the exam vivas should not present any surprises for the well-prepared candidate. The examination aims to test the knowledge of the general orthopaedic surgeon as a day 1 consultant and safety is the priority.

This book aims to give candidates the tools to answer spinal viva questions using principles, rather than to cover every potential topic in exhaustive detail. Questions are usually presented in the format of a vignette, X-ray or clinical photograph to initiate discussion. The exact format will vary from examiner to examiner and between candidates but will often start with a straightforward question that a safe candidate would be expected to address without difficulty. Subsequent questions will then test the boundaries of knowledge with further marks given for awareness of the literature and topical areas of debate.

We present key topics in a case-based format and this book can be read alone or used to supplement group revision. Differential diagnosis, interpretation of an image and management options form the key components of the majority of the scenarios.

At the end of each section, you will find a number of key references. Those in bold are the ones which we feel are essential reading for the Fellowship of the Royal College of Surgeons (FRCS) exam, with those in normal text providing further useful background reading around the topic. The 'exam tips' section gives useful information or salient points that will help maximise your score on the day.

We hope this book helps take some of the stress out of facing what may be unfamiliar scenarios!

Happy reading, keep calm and good luck!

SECTION 1
TRAUMA

1

TRAUMATIC OCCIPITO-CERVICAL INSTABILITY

You are asked to see a 34-year-old female with Down's syndrome. She presents with a 4-month history of progressive neck pain, bilateral impairment of fine motor dexterity of the hands and difficulty walking due to gait instability.

Lateral and anteroposterior (AP) plain radiographs and a computed tomography (CT) scan of the cervical spine were performed.

Q: What is the most likely diagnosis?

This patient has an acquired occipitoaxial dislocation. This is a rare diagnosis but is most seen in patients with Down's syndrome. It is most commonly asymptomatic but can be associated with pain or neurological compromise. It is classically caused by bony dysplasia or ligament and soft tissue laxity.

Plain radiographs have low sensitivity (57%) in detecting occipito-cervical (OC) injury and/or instability. The diagnosis can be most easily made using a sagittal CT scan of the cervical spine (Figure 1.2).

The power's ratio is the ratio of the distance from the posterior arch of the C1 vertebra to the basion (yellow line) divided by the distance from the anterior arch of C1 to the opisthion (red line; Figure 1.2b). A ratio of around 1 is normal. Greater than 1 indicates a possible anterior dislocation and should be correlated with the clinical presentation. A ratio of significantly less than one is indicative of an atlas (C1) ring fracture, posterior atlanto-occipital dislocation or odontoid fracture.

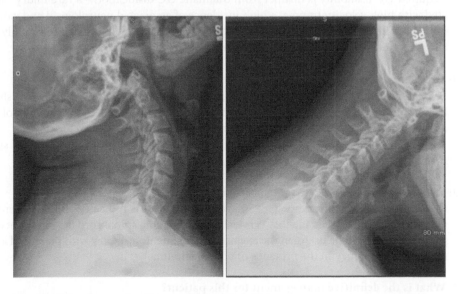

Figure 1.1   Flexion and extension X-rays of the cervical spine.

DOI: 10.1201/9781003201304-2

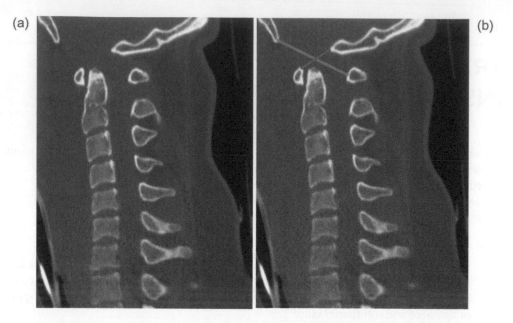

Figure 1.2   CT scan (a) (sagittal) cervical spine (b) showing occipitoaxial dissociation/dislocation.

It can be classified according to the Traynelis classification:

- Type I—Anterior occiput dislocation
- Type II—Longitudinal dislocation
- Type III—Posterior occiput dislocation

Acquired OC instability is distinct from traumatic OC dislocation—a rare injury associated with high-velocity trauma, a high incidence of associated neurological and vascular injury. It is identified in 19% of fatal cervical injuries but has become more commonly seen clinically due to improved techniques in resuscitation and imaging.

Q: How should this patient be managed?
The patient should have a detailed neurological examination and the cervical spine should be immobilised in a cervical collar if there is any history of trauma. In the presence of low- or high-energy trauma, other cervical fractures should be carefully excluded.

OC dissociation or dislocation requires urgent consult with a specialist spinal surgeon.

Q: Which other diagnostic imaging is required?
Cervical spinal magnetic resonance imaging (MRI) scan is indicated in the presence of neurological deficit. It can identify cervical disc herniation, spinal cord or nerve root compression. It can also be useful in the exclusion of ligamentous injury with preserved alignment or occult injury in the presence of possible trauma.

Q: What is the definitive management for this patient?
Surgical stabilisation is indicated for acquired OC dislocation with evidence of myelopathy or symptomatic neck pain.

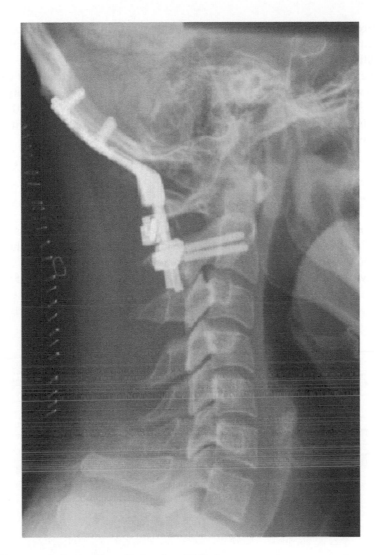

Figure 1.3 X-ray cervical spine (lateral) showing OC fusion.

This can be performed via posterior OC fusion via a midline posterior approach to the base of the skull (Figure 1.3). The patient should be positioned prone with the cervical spine securely immobilised. Fixation can be achieved via a rigid OC screw-rod or plate construct. Traction has been reported to worsen neurological compromise and so should not be attempted.

Major structures at risk include the dural venous sinuses, internal carotid artery and the vertebral artery (which runs cranially through the transverse foramen of the C2–6 vertebrae).

Exam Tips

* This is a rare condition and therefore infrequently tested. However, a working knowledge of the atlantoaxial ligamentous anatomy, as well as of the diagnosis of instability of the occipitoaxial and atlantoaxial joints is essential in clinical practice and may be

covered. Note that other causes of instability in this area include tumour, trauma and inflammatory conditions, such as rheumatoid arthritis, and these should be included in differential diagnosis.

- Remember to mention the use of Advanced Trauma and Life Support (ATLS) guidelines with any history of even minor trauma and high cervical instability!
- You should be aware of the differences between acquired and traumatic OC instability/dislocation. A detailed discussion of the surgical management of either of these is beyond the level expected of the FRCS examination.

SUGGESTED READINGS

1. Radcliff K, Kepler C, Reitman C, et al. CT and MRI-based diagnosis of craniocervical dislocations: the role of the occipitoatlantal ligament. Clin Orthop Relat Res. 2012;470(6):1602–13.
2. Panjabi M, Dvorak J, Duranceau J, et al. Three-dimensional movements of the upper cervical spine. Spine (Phila Pa 1976). 1988;13(7):726–30.

2

ATLAS FRACTURE

Q: A 45-year-old male presents to the emergency department having fallen and landed directly on his head from 2m. He suffers a concussion and complains of neck pain. Following initial assessment, he undergoes trauma CT. Please comment on this finding:

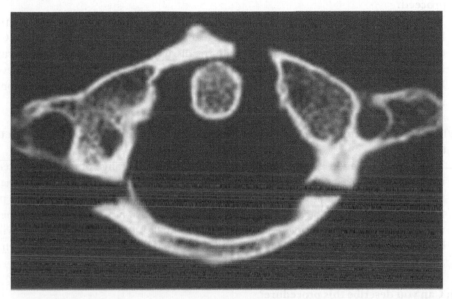

This is an axial image showing a fracture of the C1 ring. There are fractures to the anterior and posterior arches. This is a 'burst'-type injury usually because of axial loading. The eponymous name for this fracture is a Jefferson fracture.

Q: Are there any other subtypes of this fracture of which you are aware?

Gehweiler classified these fractures into 5 subtypes. Type 1 and 2 are fractures to the anterior and posterior arches and tend to be caused by hyperflexion and hyperextension mechanisms, respectively. Type 3 injuries are injuries to the anterior and posterior arches as demonstrated in this case and are sub-classified into type 3a or 3b depending upon the integrity of the transverse atlantal ligament (TAL). Type 3a injuries (intact TAL) are considered stable and type 3b injuries unstable. In type 4 injuries, the fracture extends into the lateral mass, and type 5 injuries involve the transverse process and foramen. In type 5 injuries, careful assessment with CT angiogram (CTA) should be undertaken as the vertebral artery is at risk. Most of these fractures are stable and can be managed non-operatively in a cervical orthosis.

Q: How would you assess this injury?

The stability of this type 3 injury needs to be determined and depends on the integrity of the TAL, the primary stabiliser of the upper cervical spine at the atlantoaxial junction. Spence et al. suggested that instability is indicated if the lateral mass offset—the distance between the lateral masses of C1 and C2—on an open-mouth Antero-Posterior (AP) X-ray (XR) exceeded

6.9mm², although this value has since been shown not to correlate well with TAL integrity and should be used only as a guide for assessment. Assessment on the lateral XR is by assessment of the atlanto-dens interval (ADI). This is the distance between the anterior arch of the atlas and the dens. Normally this should be <3mm and exceeding this may indicate TAL rupture.

To fully assess the integrity of the ligament, I would obtain an MRI scan. Type 3a injuries, according to the Geweiler classification, are those with an intact transverse ligament, are inherently stable, and can be managed with a cervical orthosis. However, if the ligament is ruptured this may confer instability and as such may require stabilisation.

Q: The MRI shows mid-substance disruption of the transverse ligament. How do you proceed?

This indicates that there is inherent atlanto-axial instability. Dickman classified transverse ligament injuries into type 1 (intrasubstance tear) and type 2 (bony avulsion on the C1 lateral mass). A bony avulsion associated with the disruption may heal well non-operatively in a Halo vest, which allows the bony avulsion to heal to the lateral mass. However, in light of a mid-substance tear to the ligament, I would recommend operative fixation with a C1/C2 fusion.

What is the likely consequence in terms of loss of range of motion associated with this technique?

The C1/2 articulation is particularly important for cervical range of motion. Of cervical rotation, 50% occurs at C1/2, and as such, every effort should be made to preserve the joint with a strategy of operative fixation for fracture healing with subsequent metal removal if possible. This would be a good strategy in a bony avulsion or in cases where the TAL remains intact. However, in cases of TAL rupture, this is not possible as stability will still be compromised even after bony union and primary fusion must be undertaken with appropriate patient counselling.

Q: Can you describe this procedure?

Two techniques have been described. Magerl described placing bilateral screws posteriorly from C2 across the C1/2 joint through the lateral mass of C1 and the anterior arch of C1. The technique described by Goel and Harms involves placing C1 lateral mass screws and then C2 screws which can be either pedicle screws, pars screws or laminar screws. These are then connected using a short rod on each side. Fusion can then be achieved by decorticating the C1/C2 joint and placing allograft or autograft. Care must be taken when decorticating the C/2 joint to reflect the C2 nerve cranially.

SUGGESTED READINGS

1.   Liu P, et al. 'Rule of spence' and Dickman's classification of transverse atlantal ligament injury revisited. Spine. 2019;44(5):E306–14.
2.   Spence KF, et al. Bursting atlantal fracture associated with rupture of the transverse ligament. JBJS Am. 1970;52:543–9.
3.   AO Surgery Reference: posterior C1/2 fusion.

3

ODONTOID PEG FRACTURE

Q: What does the following CT show?

The CT shows a sagittal view of a degenerate cervical spine. There is a minimally displaced fracture of C2 (the odontoid peg).

Q: What classification systems are used to describe these fractures?

The most used system is the Anderson and D'Alonzo Classification. Type I fractures are avulsion fractures of the alar ligament at the odontoid tip. Type II fractures are fractures through the waist of the odontoid, whereas type III fractures extend into the body of C2 and may involve the C1/C2 joint.

This is an Anderson and D'Alonzo Type II fracture. Eysel further classified Type II odontoid fractures. Type A are non-displaced, Type B are displaced with a fracture line from anterosuperior to posteroinferior and Type C fractures are displaced, with the fracture line from anteroinferior to posterosuperior.

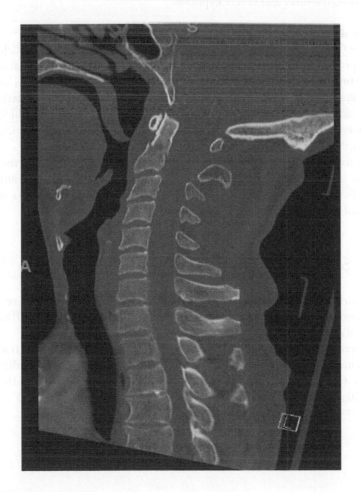

DOI: 10.1201/9781003201304-4

Q: What is the blood supply to the odontoid peg, and what significance does this have?

The base of the odontoid peg is supplied from branches of the vertebral artery whereas the apex is supplied by branches from the internal carotid artery. A vascular watershed area exists between the two areas of supply at the odontoid waist which increases non-union rates in Type II fractures.

Q: How would you manage this fracture in an elderly patient?

Odontoid fractures are the most common cervical fractures in the >65 age group. In elderly frail patients with multiple co-morbidities, I would manage this for 3 months in a cervical orthosis, accepting the likelihood of fibrous non-union. There is the potential of possible displacement with life-threatening neurological injury or development of subsequent myelopathy should further trauma be sustained.

Q: How would you manage these fractures in a young patient?

In a young patient with good bone quality and significant fracture angulation or displacement, and an Eysel type B fracture pattern, I would manage this operatively with anterior screw fixation. I would position the patient supine in a Mayfield clamp and use a minimally invasive anterior approach. I would use a cannulated 4.5mm system to place a single partially threaded screw, taking care to reach cortical bone at the odontoid tip to effect compression. Relative contraindications to this approach would include osteoporosis, Eysel type C fractures and severe kyphosis.

Q: Can you describe any other management options?

Posterior C1/C2 stabilisation using C1 lateral mass screws and C2 pedicle screws in an open approach (as described by Harms and Goel), with implant removal following bony union. This can be a useful technique in younger patients and maintains motion at C1/2. I would employ this technique when fracture morphology prevented anterior fixation, for example an Eysel type C fracture, comminuted fractures, or fractures which are unable to be reduced. This would also be a preferable technique if there were associated fractures, for example a concomitant C1 arch fracture.

Halo fixation can be applied either definitively or as a temporising measure prior to definitive internal fixation in young patients with good compliance to treatment who have no significant risk factors for non-union. In the elderly, Halo fixation is associated with significant morbidity.

SUGGESTED READINGS

1. Iyer S, Hurlbert RJ. Management of odontoid fractures in the elderly: a review of the literature and an evidence-based treatment algorithm. Neurosurgery. 2018;82(4):419–30. https://doi.org/10.1093/neuros/nyx546.
2. Gonschorek O, Vordemvenne T, Blattert T, et al. Treatment of odontoid fractures: recommendations of the Spine Section of the German Society for Orthopaedics and Trauma (DGOU). Global Spine J. 2018;8(2 Suppl):12S–17S. Published online 2018 Sep 7. https://doi.org/10.1177/2192568218768227.
3. AO Surgery reference: C2 fractures.

4

HANGMAN'S FRACTURE (BILATERAL C2 PARS FRACTURE)

Q: What does this XR show?

This is a lateral XR of the cervical spine showing an anterior spondylolisthesis of C2 (axis). This is secondary to trauma and occurs due to bilateral fractures of the pars interarticularis. The eponymous name is a 'hangman's' fracture.

Q: Can you describe the mechanism of injury?

Typically, these injuries occur because of high-energy trauma such as road traffic accidents. Hyperextension of the cervical spine leads to bilateral pars fractures. Subsequent Flexion results in tearing of the posterior longitudinal ligament and allows the intervertebral disc to sublux. Different combinations of hyperextension, flexion and axial loading lead to the different patterns of injury observed in these fractures.

Q: What imaging modalities may be useful during initial management of these injuries?

In the setting of major trauma with multiple injuries following initial resuscitation, stable patients require a trauma series CT (vertex-to-toes scanogram followed by CT

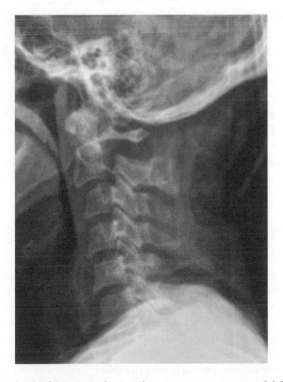

Figure 4.1   Lateral X-ray (XR) of the cervical spine showing an anterior spondylolisthesis of C2 (axis).

DOI: 10.1201/9781003201304-5

from vertex to mid-thigh) with coronal and sagittal reformats of the whole spine for fractures as well as other concomitant injuries as per National Institute for Health and Care Excellence (NICE) guidelines. If there is concern for an injury to the anterior longitudinal ligament or intervertebral disc, an MRI is mandated. Any suggestion that the fracture involves the transverse foramen mandates a CT angiogram (CTA) arch to vertex.

Q: Can you describe how these fractures are classified?

The Effendi classification system describes 3 subtypes of fracture. Type 1 fractures are minimally displaced fractures of the pars interarticularis. Type 2 fractures involve a greater degree of displacement of the anterior fragment and C2/3-disc disruption. In type 3 fractures, there is subluxation of the C2/3 facet joint.

The most used classification system, however, is that described by Levine and Edwards. It is a mechanism-based classification system comprising type I, II, IIa and III fractures. Type I fractures are the result of hyperextension and axial loading. There is minimal displacement, and the disc remains intact. Type II fractures are a result of similar hyperextension and axial loading but with additional flexion compression. The resultant fracture is both angulated and displaced, and there is a disruption to the C2/3 disc and posterior longitudinal ligament (PLL). Type IIa fractures resulting from flexion-distraction forces and have very severe angulation but no listhesis. Type III fractures result from flexion-distraction with subsequent hyperextension and result in bi-facet dislocation.

Type 1 injuries are considered stable and may be managed in a cervical orthosis or Halo immobilisation, but types II, IIa and III are considered unstable and require surgical intervention.

Q: How would you manage this injury in a 32-year-old male patient?

This is a Levine type II injury. Type II and Type III injuries are associated with significant displacement and disruption to the C2/3 intervertebral disc. These unstable injuries require operative fixation with either C2/3 ACDF or posterior C2/3 fixation using C2 pedicle screws and C3 lateral mass screws.

I would make the decision of operative approach based on the CT and MRI findings. For example, if the MRI demonstrated significant disruption to the C2/3 disc, I would perform a C2/3 ACDF to address this. However, in the absence of significant disc pathology, a posterior C2/3 fixation may sufficiently reduce and hold the fracture to effect fracture union and restore stability. If there is concern regarding the adequacy of C2/3 fixation, the construct may be extended to C1, although this will significantly compromise cervical rotation.

Q: What are the advantages and disadvantages of these different operative strategies?

The advantage of the anterior approach is that it allows one to address the disc pathology and the anterior approach has been associated with lower morbidity. The posterior approach has the advantage of giving direct access to the facet joints and therefore in type III fractures one can reduce the facet joints and fix the fracture directly. If there are concerns regarding the adequacy of fixation one has the option to extend the fixation to include C1 using lateral mass screws, although this will cause an approximate 50% loss of rotation of the cervical spine. There is currently no clear evidence in the literature supporting the superiority of one approach over the other.

Q: This fracture is deemed minimally displaced and will be managed non-operatively in a cervical orthosis. What concerns would you have for this?

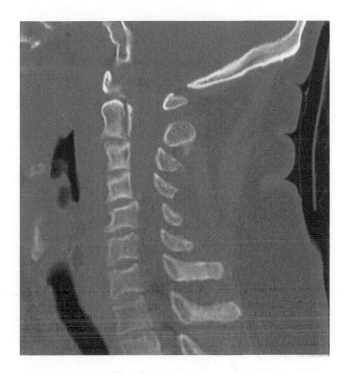

This fracture is an atypical variant as first described by Starr and Eismont. There is a coronal split extending across the posterior aspect of the vertebral body. If these fractures displace, the cord can be compressed in contrast to most of these injuries in which displacement creates more space in the canal. Some atypical fractures may extend halfway across the canal, with displacement and subsequent compression causing a Brown–Sequard syndrome. This patient should be followed up closely with regular upright X-rays and, if necessary, CT to monitor for this.

SUGGESTED READINGS

1.   Murphy H, Schroeder GD, Shi WJ, et al. Management of hangman's fractures: a systematic review. J Orthop Trauma. 2017;31:S90–5.
2.   Starr J, Eismont F. Atypical hangman's fractures. Spine. 1993;18(14):1954–7.

5

SUBAXIAL C – SPINAL FRACTURE

A 32-year-old male presents to the emergency department as a trauma call. He is immobilised in blocks and a cervical collar after a head-on road traffic collision at 60 mph (96 km/h) 1h previously. He has remained GCS 15 throughout his transportation to hospital, but complains of severe pain in his neck, numbness of both arms and significant bilateral upper limb weakness. He also has a visibly deformed left ankle which has been stabilised in a lower limb ankle splint.

He remains haemodynamically stable with a BP of 125/86 and heart rate (HR) of 86 bpm.

Q: How would you manage this patient?

This patient should be managed according to the Advanced Trauma and Life Support (ATLS) protocol, with an A–E approach. Given the high energy of the injury and reported neck pain, a cervical spinal injury must be excluded. I would perform a detailed neurological examination after giving suitable analgesia for comfort.

I would ensure that the patient's cervical spine remained immobilised in a cervical collar. I would perform a visual and manual inspection of the entire spine as well as rectal examination as part of the primary survey. I would ensure that manual inline traction was maintained when the cervical collar was removed during the logroll to inspect the posterior aspect of the cervical spine.

A trauma series CT (vertex-to-toes scanogram followed by CT from vertex to mid-thigh), with coronal and sagittal reformats, of the whole spine for fractures as well as other concomitant injuries should be requested as part of the primary survey radiographic examination. I would keep the cervical spine collar in place until imaging had been completed.

Primary survey identified no life-threatening injuries. A CT scan of his cervical spine (Figure 5.1) was completed. On detailed neurological examination, he had MRC grade 2

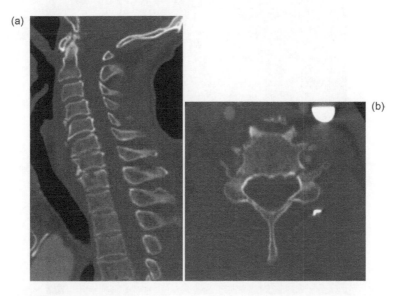

Figure 5.1 (a) Sagittal and (b) axial (slice through C6) CT scan of the cervical spine showing C6 vertebral body and bilateral pedicle fractures.

DOI: 10.1201/9781003201304-6

power below the C5 level in his arms, as well as diffuse paraesthesia bilateral in his upper limbs below shoulder height without a clearly defined dermatomal distribution. Other findings (including reflex testing) were difficult to elicit due to pain and distraction from his ankle injury.

Q: What is the diagnosis?

There is sagittal fracture of the C6 vertebral body, as well as bilateral pedicle fractures with involvement of the right transverse foramen. This is a flexion compression injury. Flexion compression/shearing fracture patterns are normally seen in the mid/lower cervical spine (specifically at C4–6). The anterior column fails in compression and the posterior column fails in tension.

They are classically associated with an antero-inferior triangular fragment ('teardrop' type; Figure 5.2) or a sagittal shear fracture of the anterior vertebral body (as in this case).

Q: Would you order any further imaging?

I would request an MRI scan of the cervical spine to exclude associated ligamentous injury, spinal instability and associated spinal cord injury (SCI).

An MRI of the cervical spine was completed. (Figure 5.3) This confirmed ligamentum flavum, anterior and posterior longitudinal ligament injury at the C5–C6 level, as well as a broad-based posterior protruding disc/osteophyte complex, chronic in appearance, causing spinal stenosis behind the C5 vertebra.

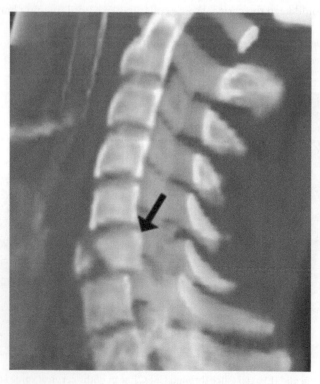

Figure 5.2   CT scan (sagittal slice) of the cervical spine showing 'teardrop' fragment of C6 vertebral body.

(a)

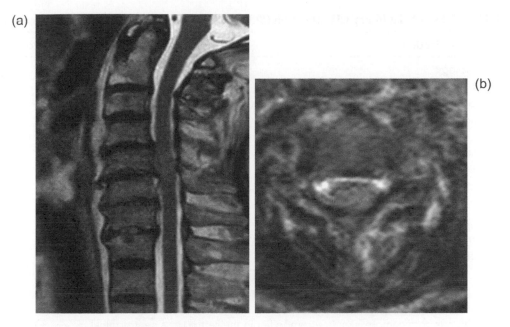

(b)

Figure 5.3 MRI scan (T2-weighted) cervical spine (a) sagittal and (b) axial (C5/6).

Q: How are these injuries classified?

Historically, the Allen–Ferguson classification was most used. It is based solely on static radiographs appearance and mechanisms of injury:

1. Flexion-compression
2. Vertical compression
3. Flexion-distraction
4. Extension-compression
5. Extension-distraction
6. Lateral flexion

The Sub-Axial Injury Classification (SLIC) Scale (Figure 5.4) is now more commonly used. It takes neurological status and posterior ligamentous complex (PLC) injury into account and informs management.

- <4—non-operative
- 4—equivocal depending on clinical judgement
- >4 surgical management

Q: How would you definitively manage this patient?

This patient has a SLIC score of >4, given the fracture morphology, neurological status and evidence of ligamentous injury on MRI. I would manage this patient surgically with a posterior decompression and instrumented fusion.

Anterior decompression, corpectomy and fusion with instrumentation are reserved for those patients with unstable burst or teardrop fractures with cord compression, as well as minimal injury to the posterior elements (not applicable in this case due to the presence of pedicle fractures).

Table 5.1 Sub-Axial Injury Classification (SLIC) Scale

SLIC Classification	Points
Morphology	–
No abnormality	0
Compression + burst	1 + 1 = 2
Distraction (e.g. facet perch or hyperextension)	3
Rotation or translation (e.g. facet dislocation, unstable teardrop or advanced-stage flexion-compression injury)	4
Disc-ligamentous complex (DLC)	
Intact	0
Indeterminate (e.g. isolated interspinous widening or MRI signal change only)	1
Disrupted (e.g. widening of the anterior disc space or facet perch or dislocation)	2
Neurological status	
Intact	0
Root injury	1
Complete cord injury	2
Incomplete cord injury	3
Continuous cord compression (neuromodifier in the setting of a neurological deficit)	+1

Early decompression (<24h) has been shown to improve long-term neurologic outcomes compared with delayed decompression (>24h).

Exam Tips

- Remember the basis of the ATLS principles (it is very worth familiarising yourself with the ATLS handbook before the exam).
- The SLIC classification is useful in that it informs management, so focus on trying to remember at least its 3 main component parts even if the individual scoring is less important for the FRCS exam.

SUGGESTED READINGS

1. Vaccaro AR, Hulbert RJ, Patel AA. The sub-axial cervical spine injury classification system: a novel approach to recognize the importance of morphology, neurology, and integrity of the disco-ligamentous complex. Spine (Phila Pa 1976). 2007;32(21):2365–74.
2. Marcon RM, Cristante AF, Teixeira WJ. Fractures of the cervical spine. Clinics (Sao Paulo). 2013;68(11):1455–61.
3. Syre P, Petrov D, Malhotra NR. Management of upper cervical spine injuries: a review. J Neurosurg Sci. 2013;57(3):219–40.

6

CERVICAL FACET FRACTURE/ DISLOCATION

A 34-year-old male presents to the emergency department (ED) after a high-velocity RTC. He is triple immobilised by the pre-hospital team, and a trauma call is initiated on arrival in the ED. He complains of severe central neck pain and left hand numbness.

Other injuries include a scalp laceration and multiple abrasions to his anterior chest wall. Focused Assessment with Sonography for Trauma (FAST) scan was negative, and he is haemodynamically stable. His GCS score is 15.

Q: What would be the initial management?

He should be managed according to Advanced Trauma and Life Support (ATLS) protocol. Given the mechanism of injury, imaging should include a chest and pelvic X-ray in the trauma bay. Trauma-series CT (vertex-to-toes scanogram followed by CT from vertex to mid-thigh) with coronal and sagittal reformats of the whole spine should be performed as per National Institute for Health and Care Excellence (NICE) guidelines (Figure 6.1).

Once a primary survey had excluded serious and life-threatening injuries, I would ensure that a secondary survey was completed to exclude extremity injuries. I would also complete a full neurological examination.

Q: What is the diagnosis?

This patient has a displaced fracture involving the right transverse process and lamina of C5. There is a unilateral right inferior C5 facet fracture, with subluxation of the right C5–C6 facet joint and associated mild (4mm) anterolisthesis (translation) of C5 relative to C6.

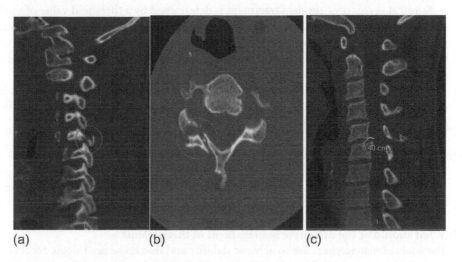

(a)   (b)   (c)

Figure 6.1 CT scan cervical spine sagittal and axial (C5/6) showing fractures to (a) inferior facet of C5, (b) C5 lamina and (c) a 4mm C5/6 spondylolisthesis.

DOI: 10.1201/9781003201304-7

Q: What are the indications for MRI in cervical facet fractures? (Figure 6.2)

MRI allows assessment of the PLC, the integrity of which is a consideration in both the SLIC and the AO Spine Subaxial Cervical Spine Classification systems.

Injuries to the PLC include the following:

- Disruption of the supraspinous and interspinous ligaments
- Posterior longitudinal ligament and posterior annulus disruption (present in 40% of unilateral dislocations and 80% of bilateral dislocations)
- Sprain or disruption of the posterior facet capsules

MRI can also identify spinal cord compression or myelomalacia and spinal cord hematoma (a poor prognostic sign for motor recovery).

Indications for an MRI scan include the following:

- Patients with acute facet dislocation with altered mental status
- Before attempting open reduction after failed closed reduction
- In the event of neurologic deterioration during closed reduction
- Any patient going to the operating room (OR) for surgical stabilisation

Timing of the MRI is controversial and depends on the severity and progression of neurologic injury. Several studies have shown that closed reduction of facet dislocations can be performed safely in awake and alert patients who can be continuously examined throughout the procedure.

Q: How can these injuries be classified?

Numerous classification schemes have been developed to characterise sub-axial cervical spine injury. The SLIC (Table 6.1) and the AO Spine Subaxial Cervical Spine Classification System, take into account morphology, discoligamentous integrity, and neurologic status.

The SLIC system and severity score identify 3 major injury characteristics (injury morphology, disc-ligamentous complex (DLC) and neurological status) with additional minor components (spinal level, anatomical osseous injury descriptors and confounders).

Surgical versus non-surgical treatment is determined by a threshold value of the SLIC severity score. If the total score is <4 (1–3), non-operative treatment is recommended. If the total is ≥5, operative treatment is recommended. This treatment may consist of reduction, neurological decompression (if indicated) and stabilisation. Cases with a total score of 4 may be treated operatively or non-operatively.

The AO Spine Subaxial Cervical Spine Classification System describes injuries based on four criteria: (1) morphology of the injury, (2) facet injury, (3) neurologic status and (4) any case-specific modifiers.

Q: What is the mechanism of facet joint fracture/dislocations?

Facet joint fracture/dislocations are flexion distraction injuries with compression across the anterior spinal column and distraction across the posterior bony elements and ligamentous complex.

Q: What should be the definitive management of this patient?

The goals of management are to achieve stability and maximise neurologic recovery. The main features to consider are therefore (1) the degree of instability of the injury, (2) the presence/absence of neurologic injury and (3) unique patient factors (e.g. comorbidities,

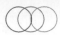
Table 6.1 Sub-Axial Injury Classification (SLIC) Scale

SLIC Classification	Points
Morphology	–
No abnormality	0
Compression + burst	1 + 1 = 2
Distraction (e.g. facet perch or hyperextension)	3
Rotation or translation (e.g. facet dislocation, unstable teardrop or advanced-stage flexion-compression injury)	4
DLC	
Intact	0
Indeterminate (e.g. isolated interspinous widening or MRI signal change only)	1
Disrupted (e.g. widening of the anterior disc space or facet perch or dislocation)	2
Neurological status	
Intact	0
Root injury	1
Complete cord injury	2
Incomplete cord injury	3
Continuous cord compression (neuromodifier in the setting of a neurological deficit)	+1

body habitus etc.) that might influence the success or failure of surgical or non-surgical treatment.

1. Unilateral facet injuries that are non-displaced or minimally displaced and without neurologic deficits are often treated non-operatively with a cervical orthosis for 6–12 weeks. Although these may seem like benign injuries, recent papers have suggested a higher rate of subsequent displacement and late chronic neck pain after non-operative management than was previously appreciated. This has prompted the question of whether some of these injuries are better treated surgically.

2. Patients with unilateral cervical facet fractures involving greater than 40% of the absolute height of the intact lateral mass or an absolute height greater than 1cm are at increased risk of failure from conservative treatment. In patients with a disc prolapse with resulting spinal cord or nerve root compression, the surgical approach should be anterior. In the absence of an anterior disc herniation, surgery can be performed from an anterior or posterior approach.

3. Patients with unilateral or bilateral facet fracture/dislocations with neurological deficits in an alert patient.

The priority in these patients is the reduction of the fracture/dislocation. Reduction should be emergent, especially in cases of bilateral dislocation. If reduction is achieved using a closed technique and the patient is immobilised in a collar, then an MRI should subsequently be obtained emergently. If MRI shows reduction and no significant compression on the spinal cord, then stabilisation should be performed on an urgent basis (within 24h).

Unilateral dislocations can be more difficult to reduce but more stable after reduction, while bilateral dislocations can be easier to reduce but less stable following reduction (because the PLL is torn).

Patients with a large disc herniation causing cord or neural element compression can be managed via an anterior approach (anterior cervical discectomy and fusion [ACDF]), while the posterior approach is appropriate for patients without an anterior disc or those fracture/dislocations that cannot be reduced either closed or via an anterior approach.

Combined anterior and posterior approaches can be used in patients with disc herniation that require anterior decompression.

Patients with unilateral or bilateral facet fracture dislocations with reduced Glasgow Coma Score (GCS)/altered mental status should **ALWAYS** have an MRI scan prior to open reduction and stabilisation. If a disc herniation is identified, closed reduction is contraindicated due to the risk of the disc being pushed into the cord, causing neurological injury. In such cases, an ACDF should be performed.

Q: What are the techniques for the reduction of displaced cervical facet fractures?

- Closed reduction of a facet dislocation as soon as possible in the emergency room setting can relieve spinal cord compression. However, traction requires analgesia and sedation, close physiologic monitoring and serial fluoroscopy. Furthermore, a closed reduction may not be possible. In our experience, the OR provides a more controlled environment for this procedure.

The commonest technique used for closed reduction of a dislocated cervical facet injury is axial traction under procedural sedation.

Technique

- Application of Gardner–Wells tongs (1 cm above the pinna and in line with the external auditory meatus and below the equator of the skull—avoids pin migration and slippage)
- Gradual increase of axial traction, with the addition of weight in 5- to 10-lb increments, adds up to 140 lb of weight or 70% body weight
- Once reduced, decrease traction weight by 10–15 lb and apply a gentle extension force to the cervical spine
- Serial neurologic exams and plain radiographs after addition of each weight addition
    - Abort if there is over-distraction of the spinal segment (>1.5 times that if the adjacent uninjured disc space)
- **Abort if neurologic exam worsens and obtain immediate MRI cervical spine**
- **Anterior cervical discectomy and fusion ± open reduction** (indicated after failed closed reduction or in the presence of an anterior disc causing cord compression seen on MRI c-spine)
    - Standard Smith–Robinson anterior cervical approach
    - Unilateral dislocations can be reduced by distracting vertebral bodies with Caspar pins and then rotating the proximal pin towards the side of the dislocation
    - Bilateral dislocations can be reduced by placing converging Caspar pins (10–20 degrees angle) and then compressing the ends together to unlock the facet joints
- Posterior instrumented stabilisation ± open reduction when closed reduction fails or is contraindicated and if open anterior reduction fails or is not required (e.g. no anterior disc prolapse)

MRI was performed to exclude a large anterior disc prolapse. This patient was managed with an ACDF performed within 24h of admission. The reduction of the spondylolisthesis and displaced facet fracture was achieved using Caspar pins inserted into the vertebral bodies of the C5 and C6 vertebrae (Figure 6.3).

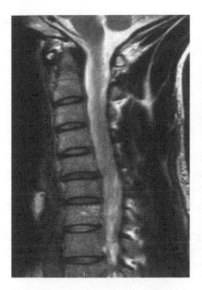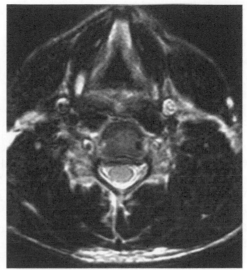

Figure 6.2   MRI scan (T2-weighted) sagittal and axial (C5/6) cervical spine. This excludes the presence of a large anterior disc prolapse/herniation.

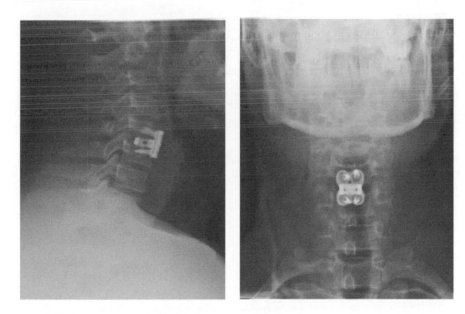

Figure 6.3   AP and lateral cervical spinal plain radiograph after C5/6 ACDF.

Exam Tip

- The key here is in the identification of the fracture, which can be best achieved by CT scan, as well as some awareness of the indications for an MRI scan. **Just to recap, in patients who are awake and cooperative, closed reduction with continuous patient monitoring is safe in the first instance.**

In obtunded/combative patients or those with distracting injuries, an MRI scan **MUST** be performed to exclude a prolapsed disc, which can be pushed into the cervical cord when a closed reduction is attempted. This would likely be a pass/fail component of this question, so it must be understood and remembered!

SUGGESTED READINGS

1. Aarabi B, Mirvis S, Shanmuganathan K, et al. Comparative effectiveness of surgical versus nonoperative management of unilateral, nondisplaced, subaxial cervical spine facet fractures without evidence of spinal cord injury. J Neurosurg Spine. 2014;20:270–7.
2. Vaccaro A, Koerner J, Radcliff KE. AOSpine subaxial cervical spine injury classification system. Eur Spine J. 2016;25(7):2173–84.
3. Patel A, Dailey A, Brodke D. Subaxial cervical spine trauma classification: the Subaxial Injury Classification system and case examples. Neurosurg Focus. 2008;25(5):E8.

7

T12 BURST FRACTURE

A 42-year-old-male is admitted after a road traffic collision (RTC).

Q: What does the imaging show?

This is a sagittal CT scan image of an AO type A4 (complete burst) fracture of the T12 vertebra. There is approximately 50% loss of vertebral body height with retropulsion of the fracture fragments. There is the suggestion of possible kyphosis cranial to this, but the scan does not extend far enough to fully assess this.

Q: On examination, the patient is neurologically intact and in significant pain. The trauma CT shows no other injuries. How would you proceed?

I would like to obtain an MRI scan to exclude posterior ligamentous complex (PLC) injury.

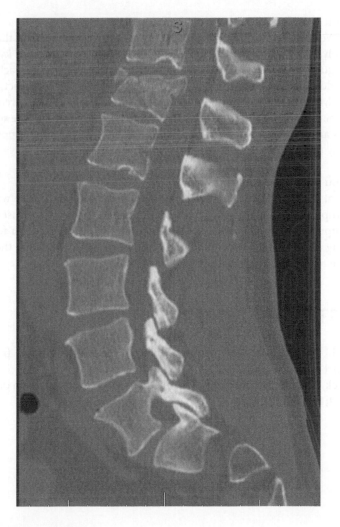

DOI: 10.1201/9781003201304-8

Q: The MRI demonstrates disruption to the ligamentum flavum, interspinous and supraspinous ligaments and bilateral facet joint effusions. How do you proceed?

I would calculate the Thoracolumbar Injury Classification and Severity Score (TLICS) score for the injury to help guide my decision-making. Using this system this patient's score is 5 (morphology 2, PLC status 3, neurology 0). I would elect to manage the fracture surgically due to the high-energy mechanism, young patient age and concern regarding stability as indicated by the significant loss of vertebral body height, extension of the fracture into the posterior elements and PLC injury. This is clearly reflected by the TLICS score.

Q: How should this patient be surgically managed?

This injury should be managed using a pedicle screw-and-rod construct. Pre-operatively I would scrutinise the CT scan to appreciate the diameter and orientation of the pedicles. In an appropriately anaesthetised and positioned patient, following level checking, I would use a direct posterior approach to the spine. Following exposure of screw entry points, I would insert pedicle screws 1 or 2 levels above and 1 or 2 levels below the fracture site. Monoaxial screws are more technically demanding to align correctly but confer greater construct stiffness and, in this young patient, would be my preferred choice.

Q: Would you consider instrumenting the fractured vertebra?

Work by Wood et al. has demonstrated that screw instrumentation at the fractured level significantly increases construct stiffness and maintains correction of kyphosis. In cases in which good purchase is obtained within the vertebral body on each side, this may spare an additional level of proximal or distal extension of the construct, sparing motion segments. McCormick et al. proposed a load sharing classification to predict failure when short segment constructs are used, based on vertebral body damage, the spread of fracture fragments and the degree of kyphosis, and these factors would be important considerations in my pre-operative planning.

Q: Would you perform a decompression?

This patient was neurologically intact pre-operatively. Although there was fracture fragment retropulsion, in a neurologically intact patient, this is not an isolated indication for decompression, and I would expect some indirect decompression following patient positioning and surgical correction of the kyphotic deformity. I would therefore not elect to perform a posterior decompression in this patient.

SUGGESTED READINGS

1. Wood K, Li W, Lebl DR, et al. Management of thoracolumbar spine fractures. Spine J. 2014;14(1):145–64.
2. McCormick T, Karaikovic E, Gaines RW. The load sharing classification of spine fractures. Spine. 1994;19(15):1741–4.

8

L1 BURST FRACTURE WITH KYPHOSIS

A 32-year-old patient is admitted following a 2m fall from a ladder.

Q: What does the imaging show?

This is a sagittal CT scan image of an incomplete burst fracture of the L1 vertebra. There is resultant kyphosis of approximately 10 degrees. Although the images above appear to demonstrate an incomplete burst injury, I would like to further scrutinise the CT to ensure no further injury to the posterior column which might indicate an unstable injury. I would look at the facet joints for evidence of subluxation or widening.

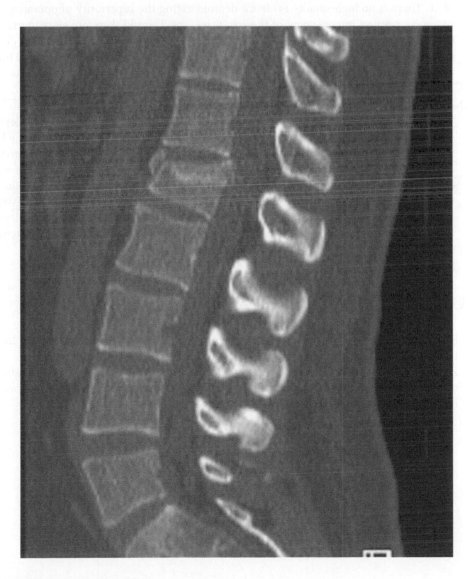

DOI: 10.1201/9781003201304-9

Q: Are you aware of any classification system pertaining to these injuries?

In 1983 Denis proposed a three-column model for spinal stability and its significance in acute thoracolumbar injuries. To the previous two-column model, he proposed a third, 'middle' column, formed by the PLL, posterior annulus fibrosus and posterior vertebral body wall. Burst fractures are anterior and middle column injuries and were suggested in this study to be unstable.

In 2005, Vaccaro et al. developed the TLICS which addressed these injuries more comprehensively. This scoring system included fracture pattern and the integrity of the PLC and neurological involvement and made recommendations as to whether they should be managed operatively or non-operatively. This was superseded in 2013 by the AO Spine Thoracolumbar Spine Injury Classification system.

Q: This patient is neurologically intact. How would you proceed?

If review of the CT revealed no further concern for posterior column injury, given that the patient is neurologically intact, the injury is stable and there is no indication for an MRI. There is no high-quality evidence demonstrating the superiority of operative versus non-operative management of these injuries, and I would therefore elect to manage this non-operatively. Following administration of appropriate analgesia, I would obtain upright X-rays to ensure that the alignment and kyphosis are still within acceptable limits when loadbearing.

Q: What degree of kyphosis would be acceptable, and why?

Various studies have shown that in the thoracolumbar spine, kyphosis of 15–30 degrees and vertebral body height loss of greater than 50% are associated with instability, which would be unacceptable, particularly in a young patient. I would not routinely prescribe a brace as studies have demonstrated an equivalence between treatment with and without bracing in these injuries. The patient could be mobilised under the supervision of the physiotherapy team and discharged with outpatient follow-up. At follow-up, I would expect repeat standing X-rays to demonstrate some progression of kyphotic deformity, but this is commonly minimal and has been shown in multiple studies not to correlate with clinical outcome.

SUGGESTED READINGS

1. Sadiqi S, Verlaan J-J, Lehr AM. Measurement of kyphosis and vertebral body height loss in traumatic spine fractures: an international study. Eur Spine J. 2017;26(5):1483–91.
2. Bailey CS, Urquhart JC, Dvorak MF, et al. Orthosis versus no orthosis for the treatment of thoracolumbar burst fractures without neurological injury: a multicentre prospective randomised equivalence trial. Spine J. 2014;14(11):2557–64.

9

CHANCE FRACTURE

A 24-year-old female presents to the emergency department after a head-on RTA at 35 mph. Primary and secondary surveys identified pain and swelling (Figure 9.1) in the thoracolumbar spine as well as seatbelt bruising over the epigastrium. She has bilaterally reduced power (Medical Research Council (MRC) grade 3+) on hip flexion, as well as paraesthesia over the anterior proximal thigh. Other examination findings are normal.

No other orthopaedic injuries are noted. Plain X-rays and CT scan of lumbar spine (Figure 9.2) are performed.

Q: How would you describe this injury?

This is a lumbar chance fracture. Chance fractures are a flexion-distraction thoracolumbar injury resulting from a failure of both the posterior and middle columns under tension, with failure of the anterior column under compression. The classical mechanism is high-velocity collision, with an anterior fulcrum such as a seatbelt. They can be bony, ligamentous or both. They are most seen in the thoracolumbar junction (T10–L2) in adults and in the lumbar spine in children. Up to 50% of cases have been associated with abdominal injuries.

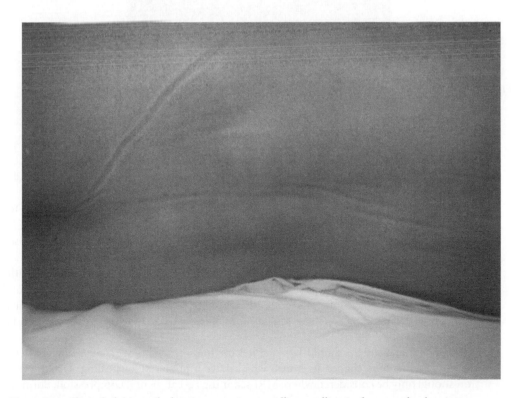

Figure 9.1 Clinical photograph showing prominent midline swelling in the upper lumbar region.

DOI: 10.1201/9781003201304-10

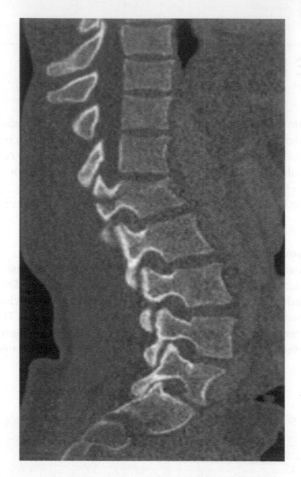

Figure 9.2   CT scan of thoracolumbar spine (sagittal view) showing fracture to L1 vertebra.

Q: Would you request any further imaging, and how should this patient be managed?

I would manage this patient according to the Advanced Trauma and Life Support (ATLS) protocol, including a thorough abdominal and genitourinary examination to exclude occult visceral injury.

Plain X-rays can be difficult to interpret in many cases, and CT scan is essential to assess the fracture pattern and degree of bony retropulsion into the spinal canal. MRI is a useful modality to identify posterior ligamentous complex (PLC) injury and can also exclude conus medullaris or spinal cord compression.

Non-operative management should be reserved for neurologically intact patients with stable fracture patterns, stable posterior elements and less than 15 degrees kyphosis. This should be with a thoracic lumbar sacral orthosis (TLSO) brace in extension for 3 months. These patients should be serially assessed radiologically to exclude progressive kyphosis and/or non-union.

Surgical management should be reserved for bony fractures with neurological deficits and ligamentous chance fractures, which have a poor rate of healing. Decompression should only be considered where MRI scanning reveals neural compression. Surgical management should be followed by a rehabilitation programme consisting of extension exercises to strengthen back muscles and reduce backache.

Q: What are the surgical approaches for this injury, and what are the potential complications?

Anterior and posterior surgical techniques have been described. Posterior approaches can be used for indirect decompression and stabilisation, either open or percutaneously. Historically, stabilisation has been three vertebral levels up and two levels down.

Improvements in pedicle screw design have made 'one-up, one-down' constructs more common. Compression can be applied across the screw heads posteriorly to close the posterior ligamentous or bony diastasis.

Complications of this procedure include pain, progressive deformity (progressive kyphosis can especially occur with occult PLL injury), flatback deformity (leading to pain and easy fatigue) and non-union.

An MRI scan was performed (not shown), which showed mild central canal stenosis secondary to a retropulsed bony fragment. Given the fracture pattern and neurological findings on examination, the patient was managed with a posterior stabalisation. Compression across the fracture site was performed to reverse the distraction forces across the posterior elements at the fractured level (Figure 9.3).

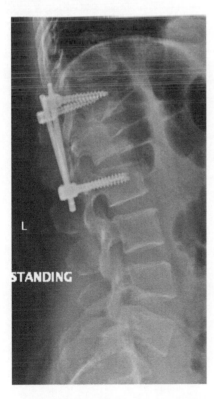
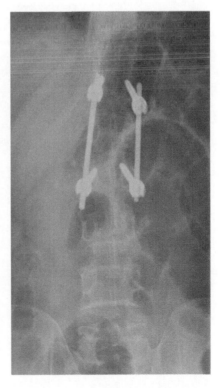

Figure 9.3   Standing X-ray thoracolumbar spine showing posterior fixation of L1 burst fracture.

SUGGESTED READINGS

1. Eismont FJ, Cuartas E. Flexion-distraction injuries of the thoracic and lumbar spine. In: Zigler JE, Eismont FJ, Garfin SR, Vaccaro AR, editors. Spine Trauma. 2nd ed. Rosemont, IL: American Academy of Orthopaedic Surgeons; 2011.

2. Liu Y-J, Chang M-C, Wang S-T. Flexion-distraction injury of the thoracolumbar spine. Injury. 2003;34(12):920–3.

3. Grossbach A, Dahdaleh N, Abel T, et al. Flexion-distraction injuries of the thoracolumbar spine: open fusion versus percutaneous pedicle screw fixation. Neurosurg Focus. 2013;35(2):E2.

10

ANKYLOSING SPONDYLITIS FRACTURE

You are called to the ED and asked to see a 51-year-old male with a known history of ankylosing spondylitis who takes infliximab. He has sustained a fall from standing height 2 days previously and complains of worsening pain in his neck. On detailed neurological examination, he has no focal neurological deficit.

Plain X-rays of the cervical spine show bridging syndesmophytes and ankylosis of the cervical and upper thoracic spine with disc space ossification but are equivocal for fracture.

A CT scan of the cervical spine is performed (Figure 10.1).

Q: What is the diagnosis?

There is a transverse fracture through the superior aspect of the C4 vertebral body. The fracture is parallel to and extends through the superior vertebral endplate and through the posterior elements with involvement of the left lamina of C4 and C5 and the distal tip of the C3 spinous process. There is no evidence of traumatic spondylolisthesis.

Q: What are the concerns around low energy spinal fractures in AS? (Table 10.1)

Spinal fractures are up to four times more common in patients with ankylosing spondylitis (AS) than the general population, with a lifetime incidence ranging from 5–15%. Most of these injuries are 3-column injuries (chalk stick fractures) resulting in an unstable spine. Many fractures pass through the intervertebral disk as opposed to the vertebral body, as the disk's elasticity is decreased, and the annulus is calcified.

They are commonly associated with an extension mechanism. Fractures can occur following even minor trauma. The susceptibility to fracture in AS after a trivial injury is due to a variety of factors. Ossification of the spinal ligaments and calcification of the annulus fibrosis alter the biomechanics of the spine, creating long lever arms limiting the ability to absorb even minor impacts. Osteoporosis stemming from stress shielding, immobility

(a)   (b)

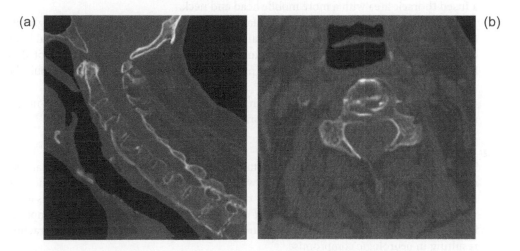

Figure 10.1   (a) Sagittal CT scan cervical spine, with (b) axial slice at C3/4 level.

DOI: 10.1201/9781003201304-11

Table 10.1 Fracture Characteristics in Ankylosing Spondylitis (AS)

	Fracture Characteristics in AS	
	Normal Spine	AS
Risk for fracture	Depends on trauma intensity	High
Intensity of injury	High intensity	Low intensity
Common site	Thoracolumbar	Cervical
Age	Young adults	Elderly
Mechanism of injury	Flexion distraction or axial compression	Hyperextension type
Unstable injury	Depends on fracture morphology	Inherently unstable
Three-column injury	Rare	Almost always
Neuro-deficit	Depends on fracture morphology	Common
Associated chest and abdominal trauma	Depends on mechanism of injury	High chance
Associated medical comorbidities	Less common	More common
Bone quality	Depending on age	Osteoporotic
Requirement of long segment fixation	Occasional	Always

and increased bony resorption also contributes to the risk of fracture for both the young and the older AS patient population. AS patients also have an amplified risk of sustaining falls due to altered gait, impaired balance and compromised horizontal gaze secondary to fixed spinal deformity. Additional risk factors for fracture in this population are advanced age, longer disease duration, progressive kyphosis and alcohol use.

There should be a low threshold for obtaining a CT scan. Fractures in AS most commonly occur in the mid-cervical and cervicothoracic junctional regions (some occur at the thoracolumbar junction). This region is particularly susceptible to injury because of oblique facet joints, proximity to the weight of the head and its location at the junction of a fused thoracic area with a more mobile head and neck.

They have a high mortality rate secondary to epidural haemorrhage, with a high rate (~75%) of neurological involvement. Spinal cord injury (SCI) can result from initial bony displacement, epidural hematoma, buckling of the ossified ligamentum flavum or disk herniation. Neurologic deficits can often present late, and therefore, patients should be admitted and observed.

The most frequent causes of death both in the acute phase and at later follow-up are respiratory complications such as pneumonia.

Q: How should this patient be managed?

This 3-column injury represents an unstable fracture and warrants surgical management. A multidisciplinary team approach with a thorough pre-operative plan is essential. Patients may have pre-existing pulmonary disease requiring evaluation and optimisation. The anaesthesia team should be aware of any cervical kyphotic deformity; attempts to hyperextend the neck will either be restricted or will cause extension through the fracture resulting in neurologic compromise.

Fibre-optic intubation may be required.

A detailed neurological examination should be performed. The surgical approach depends on patient characteristics as well as fracture location and pattern. Surgical positioning may need to be modified to accommodate for spinal deformity. Stable fractures without neurological compromise can be managed with **immobilisation in the existing kyphotic position, admission for observation and MRI scan of the cervico-thoracic spine**.

Pre-operative evaluation of the fracture pattern using both an MRI and CT scan of the affected area must be performed. This is to assess for posterior ligamentous restraint, neurologic compression and function and bone quality.

Spinal decompression with instrumented fusion is indicated in patients with unstable fracture patterns and neurologic compromise. The aim of this procedure is the stabilisation of the fracture and decompression of neurological structures, but deformity correction should not be attempted. Multiple points of fixation above and below the fracture are necessary in patients with AS. Osteoporosis and long lever arms of the ankylosed spine increase the forces on the pedicle screws around the fracture site.

Exam Tips

- It is easy to focus on the spinal fracture itself in this case. However, recognition of the other challenges associated with AS, including likely difficulties with intubation and patient positioning, are key to showing that you are not just giving a generic, memorised answer.
- Always get a CT scan in AS patients with neck pain. Fractures can occur with minimal trauma and can be difficult to visualise on X-ray.
- Regarding fracture management itself in AS fractures, the key difference should be the use of a longer construct than the traditional 'two up–two down' construct employed in other cases.

SUGGESTED READINGS

1. Lukasiewicz AM, Bohl DD, Varthi AG. Spinal fracture in patients with ankylosing spondylitis: cohort definition, distribution of injuries, and hospital outcomes. Spine (Phila Pa 1976). 2016;41(3):191–6.
2. Chaudhary SB, Hullinger H, Vives MJ. Management of acute spinal fractures in ankylosing spondylitis. ISRN Rheumatol. 2011;2011:150484.

11

DISH (FORESTIER DISEASE) FRACTURES

A 64-year-old carpenter presents to the ED after a fall from standing height. He has a long-standing history of pain and stiffness in his cervical spine. He complains of some left arm numbness and mild weakness which on clinical assessment matches the C7 dermatome and myotome. Medical history includes diabetes mellitus type 2 and hypercholesterolaemia.

Plain X-ray, CT scan (Figure 11.1) and MRI scan (Figure 11.2) of the cervical spine are performed.

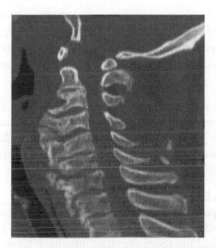
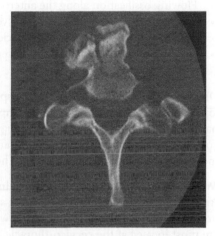

Figure 11.1   CT scan cervical spine sagittal and axial (C6/7) showing multiple bridging osteophytes across the cervical spine and a vertically orientated fracture of the C7 vertebra.

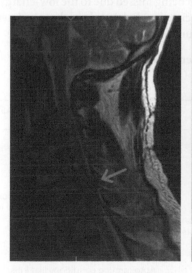
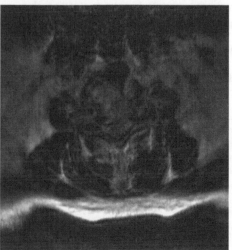

Figure 11.2   MRI scan (T2-weighted) cervical spine sagittal and axial (C6/7) showing possible disruption of the ligamentum flavum at the C6/7 level.

DOI: 10.1201/9781003201304-12

Q: What is the likely diagnosis?

The underlying diagnosis is diffuse idiopathic skeletal hyperostosis (DISH). There are non-marginal syndesmophytes from C2 to T1. The disc spaces remain preserved and non-ossified, which differentiates this condition from ankylosing spondylitis (AS) (Table 11.1).

CT scan cervical spine shows a vertically orientated fracture of the C7 vertebra with extension into both the superior and the inferior endplate. The MRI scan shows no spinal cord signal change; however, there is possible ligamentum flavum disruption at the injured level (red arrow), along with increased signal intensity within the disk spaces of C6–7 and C7–T1. Extensive oedema of the posterior soft tissues with extension into the interspinous spaces at C5–C6 and C6–C7 represents likely interspinous ligaments injury.

Q: How can DISH be diagnosed and what are its associated conditions?

Diagnostic criteria of DISH are as follow:

- Flowing ossification along the anterolateral aspect of at least 4 contiguous vertebrae
- Preservation of disc height in the involved vertebral segment; relative absence of significant degenerative changes (e.g., marginal sclerosis in vertebral bodies or vacuum phenomenon)
- Absence of facet-joint ankylosis; absence of SI joint erosion, sclerosis or intraarticular osseous fusion

DISH is an ankylosing disorder of the spine characterised by ossification of the anterior longitudinal ligament and can be accompanied by ossification of the posterior longitudinal and extraspinal ligaments. Its aetiology is unknown, but it is associated with older age, gout, obesity and type 2 diabetes. Large anterior osteophytes can cause decreased range of motion in the spine, dysphagia, stridor, hoarseness and sleep apnoea.

Q: What is the pathogenesis of fractures in DISH?

Ankylosis of spinal segments causes the spine to lose mobility and to function like a long bone. As a result, fractures can occur with minimal trauma (similar to AS). Fractures are most located at the cervico-thoracic and the thoracolumbar junctions. Neurological injury is associated more commonly with fractures in the cervical spine than the thoracic spine, as the rib cage and sternum are a stabilising force in the thoracic spine.

Fractures associated with DISH are at risk of being missed due to the low-energy mechanism of injury. Delayed diagnosis can be associated with delayed paralysis and neurological compromise, particularly in cervical fractures.

Q: What are the radiological differences between DISH and AS?

Table 11.1 Characteristics of DISH and AS

	Diffuse Idiopathic Skeletal Hyperostosis (DISH)	Ankylosing Spondylitis (AS)
Aetiology	Idiopathic	Autoimmune
Incidence	2.9-25%	0.05-1.4%
Age of onset	> 45 years	<30 years
Sex ratio (M/F)	2:1	3:1
Clinical features	Pain, radiculopathy, dyshagia, risk of spinal and peripheral fractures	Pain, spinal stiffness, postural abnormalities, involvement of large periphheral joints
Radiological features	Affects anterior longitudinal ligaments of the spine, spares IV discs and SI joints	Intervertebral jont fusion, especially the SI joints
Lab Investigations	Non specific and inconclusive	High ESR and CRP, presence of HLA-B27 (in most cases)
Associated diseases	Obesity, DM, Hypervitaminosis A	Autoimmune conditions like iritis, uveitis, ulcerative colitis,
Treatment	Symptomatic	DMARDS, NSAIDS, surgery (occasionally)

Q: How should this patient be managed?

The patient should be placed in a cervical collar to stabilise the cervical spine. Many fractures without neurological compromise or instability can be managed definitively with **activity modification, physical therapy, brace wear, non-steroidal anti-inflammatory drugs (NSAIDs) and bisphosphonate therapy**.

However, **the soft tissue injury and neurological compromise in this patient warrant surgical decompression, and stabilisation is indicated**.

As with all cases of surgical management of the unstable cervical spine, care should be taken to position the patient using C-spine precautions onto a radiolucent Jackson table. The head should be pinned using Mayfield pins (Figure 11.3) which are then attached using the adaptor to the Jackson table, keeping the neck in a neutral position. The patient is then 'sandwiched' into place and turned using the Jackson turning frame into a prone position.

Laminectomy is performed to decompress the spinal cord and posterior stabilisation is achieved using pedicular and/or lateral mass screws depending on the level of fixation (Figure 11.4).

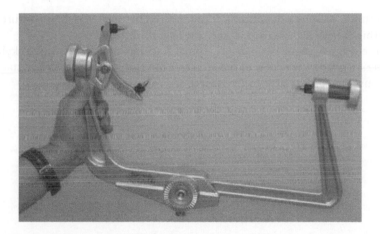

Figure 11.3   The Mayfield skull clamp.

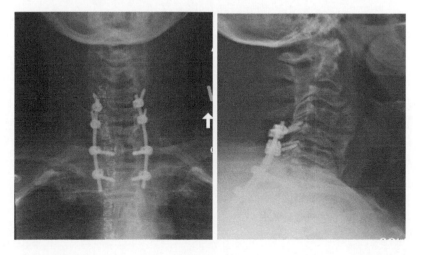

Figure 11.4   AP and lateral cervical spine X-ray after posterior decompression and fixation of sub-axial vertebral fracture.

Exam Tips

- DISH is an easily examined topic and so you should be able to answer on it in detail. Patients with DISH who present with trivial trauma should be assessed by 3-dimensional imaging without delay, even when there are no immediate neurological symptoms, to prevent a missed or delayed diagnosis. You should particularly be aware of the radiological distinctions between AS and DISH, as outlined above.
- Remember: A major risk of screw insertion in the sub-axial spine is injury to the vertebral arteries. The vertebral arteries arise from the subclavian arteries, one on each side of the body, and then enter deep to the transverse process at the level of the 6th cervical vertebrae (C6), or occasionally (in 7.5% of cases) at the level of C7. They then proceed superiorly, in the transverse foramen of each cervical vertebra to C2.

SUGGESTED READINGS

1. Murakami Y, Mashima N, Morino T. Association between vertebral fracture and diffuse idiopathic skeletal hyperostosis. Spine. 2019;44(18):E1068–74.
2. Westerveld LA, Verlaan JJ, Oner FC. Spinal fractures in patients with ankylosing spinal disorders: a systematic review of the literature on treatment, neurological status and complications. Eur Spine J. 2009;18(2):145e56.

12

SACRAL FRACTURES

A 47-year-old male presented to the ED after a fall from a 3-storey height in an apparent suicide attempt. The patient was managed according to Advanced Trauma and Life Support (ATLS) protocol.

Plain radiograph of the chest and pelvis (Figure 12.1), as well as a cervical spinal and head CT scan, was performed as part of a trauma series evaluation. Primary and secondary survey revealed multiple injuries including bilateral rib fractures, a small subdural haematoma, bilateral haemathoraces.

Q: What does Figure 12.1show?

This AP plain X-ray of the pelvis shows comminuted and displaced fractures of the right superior and inferior pubic rami, with suspected intra-articular extension to the anterior wall of the right acetabulum. The sacrum is challenging to assess given overlying bowel gas right sacral alar fracture.

Q: What further investigations should be ordered?

Radiographs only show 30% of sacral fractures. Lateral X-rays can be an effective screening tool for sacral fractures but are not part of the standard ATLS primary survey imaging.

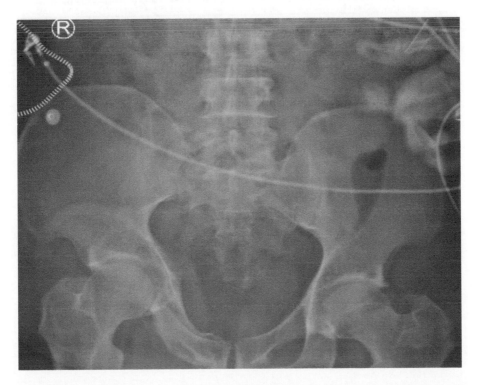

Figure 12.1   AP pelvic X-ray showing comminuted and displaced right pubic ramus and acetabular fracture.

DOI: 10.1201/9781003201304-13

Inlet and outlet pelvic X-rays (Figure 12.2) should be taken in the radiographic investigation of sacral fractures. The inlet view allows the best assessment of sacral spinal canal and superior view of S1, while the outlet view provides true AP of the sacrum.

Coronal and sagittal reconstructions of pelvic CT scans are the diagnostic study of choice (Figure 12.3). MRI scans of the lumbar spine and pelvis are recommended when neural compromise is suspected.

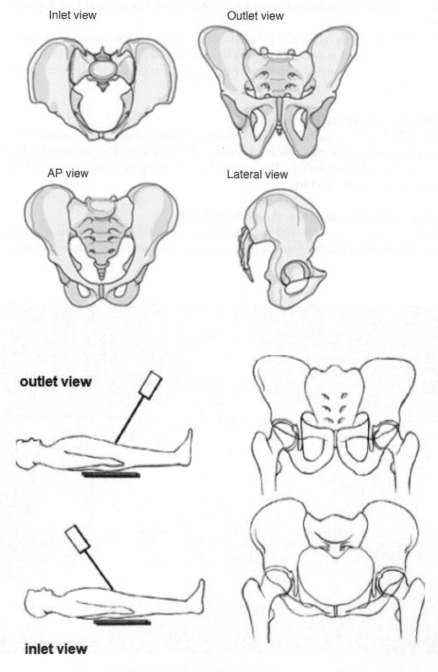

Figure 12.2   Inlet and outlet radiographic views of the pelvis.

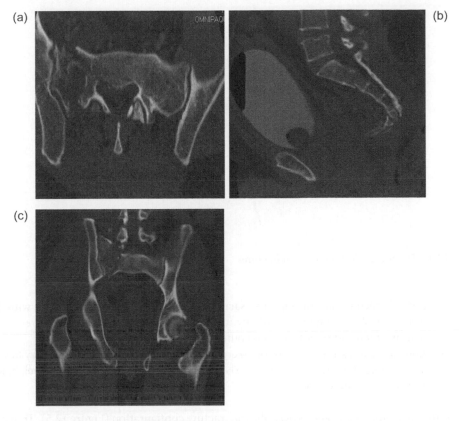

Figure 12.3 CT scan pelvis (clockwise from top left): (a) axial, (b) sagittal and (c) coronal.

Q: What do Figures 12.3a–c show?

Figure 12.3 shows axial, sagittal and coronal slices through a CT scan of the pelvis. It shows a displaced and comminuted right sacral ala fracture, extending inferiorly into the left sacral alar and coccyx with extension into the neural foramina. The coronal slice (Figure 12.3c) shows the superior translation of the right sacral ala.

There is superior displacement of the lateral sacral fracture. This likely represents a vertical shear-type pelvic injury. There is also a left L5 transverse process fracture. (L4 and L5 transverse process fractures can commonly be associated with vertical shear-type sacral fractures, particularly after high-velocity injuries.)

Q: What is the clinical relevance of injury to the lower sacral nerve roots (S2–5)?

The lower sacral nerve roots (S2–S5) have a role in maintaining anal sphincter tone/voluntary contracture and perianal sensation. Unilateral preservation of nerves is adequate for bowel and bladder control.

Q: How can sacral fractures be classified?

There are several classification systems for sacral fractures. The Denis classification (Figure 12.4) is the most frequently used.

- Zone 1 fractures are lateral to foramina. They are most common (50%), with a low incidence of nerve injury (5%). Nerve injuries in these fractures usually occur to L5 nerve root which lies on the cranial aspect of the sacral ala.

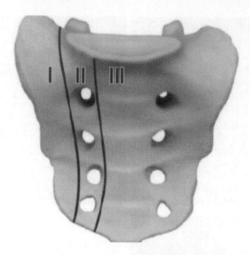

Figure 12.4 Denis classification of sacral fractures.

- Zone 2 fractures are through the sacral foramen. They may be unstable, with fractures with shear components highly unstable. Unstable fractures have increased risk of non-union and poor functional outcome.
- Zone 3 fractures are medial to the sacral foramina into the spinal canal. They have the highest rate of neurologic deficit (60%) with a significant incidence of bowel, bladder and sexual dysfunction.

Other fracture classifications describe the fracture configuration (Figure 12.5). Transverse and U-shaped sacral fractures also have a high incidence of nerve dysfunction. U-type sacral fractures result from axial loading and represent spino-pelvic dissociation.

Q: How can this injury be definitively managed?

Management of sacral fractures is dependent on fracture configuration, patient factors and neurological status. Non-operative management with progressive weight-bearing is indicated in patients with <1cm displacement and no neurologic deficit or those with insufficiency fractures.

Surgical management is indicated for in patients with

- displaced fractures >1cm,
- soft tissue compromise,
- persistent pain after non-operative management and
- displacement of fracture after non-operative management.

Decompression of neural elements is indicated in patients with neurological symptoms and can be achieved posteriorly with a laminectomy.

The fracture in this case is significantly comminuted with vertical displacement, representing instability. This can be managed in the first instance using pelvis external fixation via AIIS screws. These provide early stabilisation while the patient is being medically optimised, particularly if the patient requires other urgent interventions.

The external fixation pins can also help in reduction of the displaced fracture at the time of definitive fixation. Sagittal plane fractures can be managed percutaneously with sacro-iliac, trans-sacral (Figure 12.6) or trans-iliac trans-sacral screws. **The major structure**

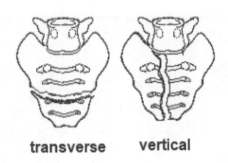

transverse   **vertical**

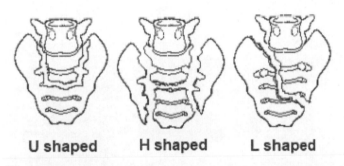

U shaped   **H shaped**   **L shaped**

Figure 12.5   Sacral fracture configuration.

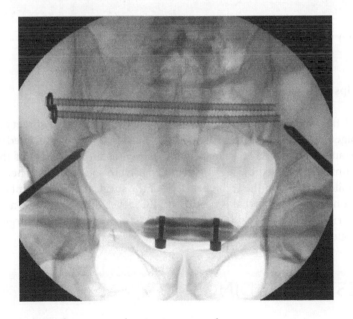

Figure 12.6   Intraoperative fluoroscopy showing trans-sacral screws.

at risk is the L5 nerve root. In the presence of significant instability or spino-pelvic disso-ciation, sacral screws can be augmented by lumbo-pelvic fixation (Figure 12.7) to maxim-ise stiffness and reduce the rate of screw failure. Lumbo-sacral fixation classically involves the use of pedicle screws into the lumbosacral spine, with pelvic fixation using S2 alar-iliac (S2AI) screws or iliac screws.

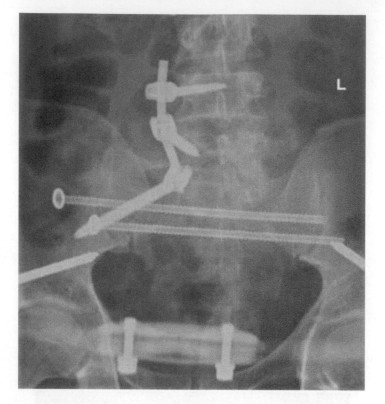

Figure 12.7 X-ray (AP) showing lumbopelvic fixation.

Exam Tips

- Sacral fractures fall under the umbrella of pelvic and spinal surgery and may need management by both subspecialties. These injuries are often associated with significant polytrauma and so ATLS management, as well as an awareness of the use of damage-control orthopacdics (DCO) should be used in a good answer here.
- A detailed answer on the technical steps of the surgical management of these injuries is beyond the scope of what is needed at FRCS level, but you should certainly be aware of the risk of neurological injury and the fractures that warrant surgical, rather than non-operative, management.

SUGGESTED READINGS

1. Beckmann NM, Chinapuvvula NR. Sacral fractures: classification and management. Emerg Radiol. 2017;24(6):605–17.
2. Robles LA. Transverse sacral fractures. Spine J. 2009;9(1):60–9.
3. Bishop JA, Dangelmajer S, Corcoran-Schwartz I, et al. Bilateral sacral ala fractures are strongly associated with lumbopelvic instability. J Orthop Trauma. 2017;31(12):636–9.

13

NEUROGENIC SHOCK

A 29-year-old man presents as a trauma call in the ED of your major trauma centre (MTC) after a neck injury sustained 4h previously, after diving headfirst into a shallow pool. He was triple immobilised at the scene.

A primary survey was completed. The patient is GCS 12 (E3, V4, M5).

Haemodynamic observations are as follows: BP 78/45 heart rate (HR): 46 (regular) Temp: 36.1 °C

On examination, no motor or sensory function was noted below the C5 level. No voluntary anal contraction (VAC) was noted, but the bulbocavernosus reflex is intact.

An urgent trauma series CT scan (Figure 13.1) was performed.

Q: What is the likely cause of the patient's bradycardia and hypotension?

This patient is likely to have a complete spinal cord injury (SCI) related to an injury at the C5 level. His haemodynamic compromise with the pattern of injury is likely to be a sign of neurogenic shock. The presence of the bulbocavernosus reflex excludes spinal shock.

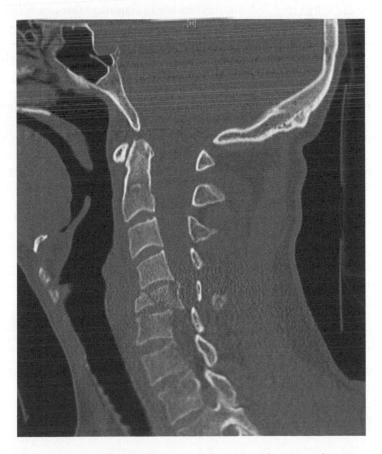

Figure 13.1   CT scan cervical spine (sagittal) showing a fracture to the C5 vertebra.

DOI: 10.1201/9781003201304-14

Other causes of circulatory shock classically cause hypotension and tachycardia rather than bradycardia and hypotension.

Q: What is the pathogenesis of this condition?

Neurogenic shock occurs when the spinal cord is injured. Cardiac sympathetic innervation and vasomotor tone are lost, while parasympathetic innervation from the vagus nerve remains intact.

This results in **hypotension and bradycardia**, the classical signs of **neurogenic shock**. This contrasts with spinal shock, which occurs within 24h of SCI and leads to a total loss of reflexes, flaccid paralysis and complete sensory loss below the level of injury.

Preganglionic sympathetic neurons originating in the hypothalamus, pons and medulla are in the intermediolateral cell column of the spinal cord between the first thoracic (T1) and second lumbar (L2) vertebrae. Theoretically, any SCI within or above this could cause sympathetic disruption. Sympathetic innervation of the heart only occurs from T1 to T5, neurogenic shock classically only occurs when the lesion is above the mid-thoracic (T6) level.

Q: What is the immediate management of this patient?

Early identification of neurogenic shock is key. The aim is to maintain perfusion to the body and compromised spinal cord, helping reduce secondary cord damage.

One characteristic of neurogenic shock is the partial resistance to fluids, which could be misinterpreted as volume loss. This could result in overhydration of the patient, causing pulmonary or spinal cord oedema. Appropriate management involves initial use of fluids followed by Swan-Ganz monitoring for careful fluid management and support of HR and blood pressure (BP) by vasopressors and sympathomimetics. The identification of neurogenic shock followed by appropriate treatment and maintenance of BP are interventions linked with better neurological outcome.

Q: What are the other possible cardiorespiratory sequelae because of this injury?

High cervical SCI is associated with respiratory compromise due to the diaphragmatic innervation by the C3, 4, 5 nerve roots. This is characterised by low lung volumes and a weak cough secondary to respiratory muscle weakness. Autonomic dysfunction and early-onset sleep-disordered breathing can compound this respiratory compromise.

Paralysis of the intercostal muscles creates an unstable chest wall such that during inspiration, the negative intrathoracic pressure causes paradoxical inward depression of the ribs. This results in increased work of breathing, and a tendency towards distal airway collapse and micro-atelectasis. Airway secretions may accumulate in the lungs through increased production or decreased clearance.

Patients are vulnerable to respiratory illnesses in the first year after injury but continue to suffer from respiratory complications throughout life.

SUGGESTED READINGS

1. Taylor MP, Wrenn P, O'Donnell AD. Presentation of neurogenic shock within the emergency department. Emerg Med J. 2017;34(3):157–62.
2. Ruiz IA, Squair JW, Phillips AA. Incidence and natural progression of neurogenic shock after traumatic spinal cord injury. J Neurotrauma. 2018;35(3):461–6.

14

SPINAL SHOCK

A 61-year-old man presents to the ED after a 30ft fall from a ladder while working on a construction site. A CT scan and an MRI scan (Figure 14.1) are completed. Medical history includes diabetes mellitus Type 2 and poorly controlled hypertension.

On examination, the patient is GCS 15 with flaccid tone in his lower limbs and a complete loss of motor and sensory function below the level of the injury (T5). Deep tendon reflexes of the lower limb (knee-jerk and ankle-jerk) are absent. The bulbocavernosus reflex is also absent.

On admission, BP: 115/70 heart rate (HR): 62 T: 37.8

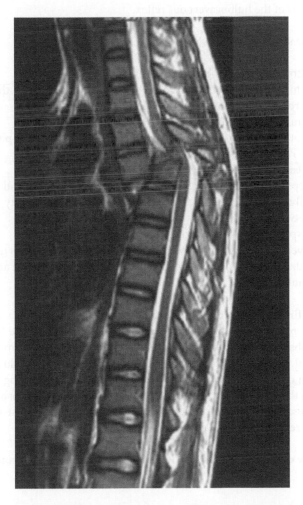

Figure 14.1 Sagittal view MRI scan (T2 weighted) (image of thoracolumbar spine) showing dislocation of T5/6, with spondyloptysis of T4 over T5 and a fracture of the T5 vertebra. Spinal cord contusion and severe cord compression at the level of the injury also noted.

DOI: 10.1201/9781003201304-15

Q: What are the causes of the patient's examination findings?
The most likely diagnosis is spinal shock. This is a sudden and reversible loss of neuro-logical function, including reflexes, rectal tone, and muscle tone below the level of an acute spinal cord injury (SCI). It is characterised by flaccid areflexic paralysis, bradycardia, hypotension (due to a loss of sympathetic tone) and an absent bulbocavernosus reflex (characterised by involuntary anal sphincter contraction in response to squeezing the glans penis/clitoris or tugging on an indwelling Foley catheter).

While this patient has a 'normal' blood pressure (BP) using standard physiological parameters, given his history of uncontrolled hypertension, his reading may represent a relative hypotension when compared with his normal baseline.

Q: What is this patient's American Spinal Cord Injury Association (ASIA) score?
Neurological status cannot be evaluated until the patient is out of the initial phase of spinal shock (i.e., the bulbocavernosus response has returned or at least 48h has elapsed since the injury).

The latter is important to note because conus or cauda equina injuries may lead to permanent loss of the bulbocavernous reflex.

Q: What are the stages of spinal shock?

- Phase I: areflexia/hyporeflexia (0–1 day)
  During this period, cutaneous (polysynaptic) reflexes such as the bulbocavernosus and the cremasteric reflex begin to recover.
- Phase 2: initial reflex return (1–3 days)
  Polysynaptic reflexes return and become stronger during this phase; monosynaptic (patellar) remain absent.
- Phase 3: early hyper-reflexia (4 days to 1 month)
  Most deep tendon reflexes first reappear during this period, and they are evident in almost all subjects within 30 days. There is significant variability in the rate of reflex return between individuals.
- Phase 4: spasticity/hyper-reflexia (1–12 months)
  The delayed plantar response (see the following discussion) has disappeared in most cases. Cutaneous and deep tendon reflexes become hyperactive and respond to min-imal stimuli.

Q: What is the first reflex to return after the onset of spinal shock?
A pathologic reflex, the delayed plantar reflex (DPR), is usually the first reflex to return and can be observed within hours of injury. In most cases, it is transient and disappears within several weeks. The DPR requires an unusually strong stimulus, in contrast to the Babinski sign or normal plantar response, and is elicited by stroking a blunt instrument upward from the heel toward the toes along the lateral sole of the foot and then continuing medially across the volar aspect of the metatarsal heads. In response to the stimulus, the toes flex and relax in a delayed sequence.

Q: What are the differences among spinal shock, neurogenic shock and hypovolaemic shock?

Table 14.1 **Differences among Spinal, Neurogenic and Hypovolaemic Shock**

	Spinal Shock	Neurogenic Shock	Hypovolaemic Shock
BP	Hypotension	Hypotension	Hypotension
HR	Bradycardia	Bradycardia	Tachycardia
Reflexes/ bulbocavernosus reflex	Absent	Variable/independent	Variable/independent
Motor	Flaccid paralysis	Variable/independent	Variable/independent
Time	48–72h immediately after SCI	~48–72h immediately after SCI	excessive blood loss
Mechanism	Peripheral neurons become temporarily unresponsive to brain stimuli.	Disruption of autonomic pathway leads to loss of sympathetic tone and decreased systemic vascular resistance.	Decreased preload leads to decreased cardiac output (Starling's law).

Q: How can this injury be managed?

Treatment of SCIs begins at the accident scene with proper spinal immobilisation, which should include a rigid cervical collar and transport on a firm spine board with lateral support devices. The patient should be rolled with standard logroll techniques with control of cervical spine. Spine boards should be used for transport only, and patients should be removed when clinically safe, as decubitus ulcers can occur after only 30–60 minutes on a backboard.

Initial medical management should include deep vein thrombosis (**DVT**) **prophylaxis, except when contraindicated in the setting of suspected major haemorrhage or a history of coagulopathy.** Careful haemodynamic monitoring and stabilisation are critical in early treatment.

The evidence surrounding the use of high-dose methylpredisone after SCI is mixed. Current guidelines recommend against administration due to a risk of complications and lack of evidence as to their clinical benefit. Similarly, some studies have recommended systemic and local hypothermia for acute traumatic SCI. However, the evidence for this is currently weak, and it is not currently recommended due to the risk of complications, including sepsis and coagulopathy.

Management of incomplete SCI frequently involves surgical decompression when the patient hits a neurologic plateau or if worsens neurologically. This may facilitate nerve root function return at level of injury (may recover 1–2 levels).

Management of most complete SCI involves stabilising the spine to facilitate rehabilitation and minimise the need for Halo or orthosis. Decompression may lead to some neurological benefit.

Q: What is the prognosis of complete versus incomplete SCI?

- Complete injuries: improvement of one nerve root level can be expected in 80% of patients, improvement of two nerve root levels can be expected in 20% of patients.
- Incomplete injuries: variable; patients who show more rapid recovery have a better prognosis; when recovery plateaus, it rarely resumes improvement.

Exam Tip

- For obvious reasons, you will not be faced with one of these patients as a clinical case. However, an understanding of the differences between neurogenic and spinal shock, as well as the calculation of the ASIA score, are the key learning points for this case.

SUGGESTED READINGS

1. Ditunno JF, Little JW, Tessler A. Spinal shock revisited: a four-phase model. Spinal Cord. 2004;42(7):383–95.
2. Ko H-Y. Revisit spinal shock: pattern of reflex evolution during spinal shock. Korean J Neurotrauma. 2018;14(2):47–54.

15

TRANSIENT QUADRIPLEGIA AND RETURN TO SPORT

A 21-year-old semi-professional rugby player is admitted to the ED as a trauma call after a head-on collision during a tackle. He presents to hospital triple immobilised and on a spinal board. He reports an immediate loss of sensation and significant bilateral upper and lower limb weakness after the incident.

The 90-minute interval since the incident has seen a gradual improvement in neurological symptoms. At the time of review in the trauma bay, the patient is moving his arms and legs freely and has bilaterally normal neurological findings in the arms and legs on detailed assessment.

Q: What is the likely diagnosis?

The most likely diagnosis is transient quadriplegia (TQ).

Clinical presentation includes bilateral sensory changes, motor changes, or combined sensorimotor deficits. The symptoms occur in either both arms, both legs or both arms and legs. Symptoms range from mild to severe and total body numbness may occur. Burning paraesthesia may be present in the cervical region. Neck pain is classically absent. Weakness can range from mild to complete paralysis. The symptoms of TQ are, by definition, transient and usually last less than 15 minutes but may last up to 48h. If symptoms last longer, it cannot be TQ, and another diagnosis should be considered.

TQ most commonly occurs because of axial loading of the spine. In athletes with narrowing of the anterior-posterior (AP) diameter of the spinal canal, both hyperextension and hyperflexion can lead to cord compression. This is referred to as the 'pincer mechanism'.

Q: How would you proceed with further investigation of this patient?

CT scan of the cervical spine should be ordered as part of the trauma series. If no fracture is identified despite significant neck pain, cervical flexion/extension X-rays can be obtained to exclude ligamentous instability.

MRI scans of the cervical spine are performed to evaluate patients with TQ, even if symptoms have completely resolved. The MRI is required to rule out a herniated disc, spinal stenosis or spinal cord contusion.

The Torg ratio describes a radiographic method of determining the presence of cervical canal stenosis on plain radiographs of the cervical spine. It compares the AP dimension of the vertebral canal to that of vertebral body; ratio = a/b. (Figure 15.1) A ratio of one is considered normal and a ratio of <0.80 is 'significant spinal stenosis'.

In cases of persistent neurologic deficit, such as arm and/or leg weakness or numbness, an electromyography and nerve conduction velocity (EMG/NCV) test may be ordered. EMG/NCV tests are useful to determine which nerve is affected and how severely it is damaged or irritated.

DOI: 10.1201/9781003201304-16

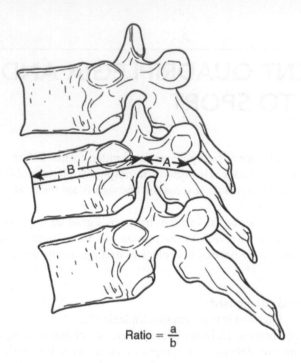

Ratio = $\dfrac{a}{b}$

Figure 15.1   Torg ratio.

Q: What are the current recommendations concerning return to play (RTP) in this case?

Exact RTP criteria are controversial. An athlete that is still symptomatic or has positive neurologic findings on examination should not return to competition. Other reasons to absolutely prevent an athlete from returning to play are ligamentous instability, a single injury with evidence of spinal cord damage on MRI scan (myelomalacia), more than one event of TQ, an upper cervical spinal anatomical abnormality (such as odontoid hypoplasia, os odontoideum and atlantooccipital fusion) and/or symptoms lasting longer than 48h.

Ligamentous instability has been defined as 'more than 11° of angulation or 3.4 mm translation between two adjacent vertebrae on flexion/extension radiographs'[2]. Recurrence rate is high in the athletes who have experienced one episode of TQ. The athlete and their family should be made aware of this risk, and patient counselling of the patient and family is key.

SUGGESTED READINGS

1.   Torg JS, Pavlov H. Cervical spinal stenosis with cord neurapraxia and transient quadriplegia. Clin Sports Med. 1987;6(1):115–33.
2.   Fagan K. Transient quadriplegia and return-to-play criteria. Clin Sports Med. 2004;23(3):409–19.

Section 2
DEGENERATIVE SPINAL CONDITIONS

16

CERVICAL RADICULOPATHY

A 67-year-old male presents with a month-long history of recurrent right 4th/5th finger numbness and pain. He is normally fit and well and works as a carpenter. His medical history is positive for hypertension, and he had a 30-pack year smoking history.

On examination, he has right-sided weakness of little finger flexion, as well as reduced sensation in the C8 dermatome. He had no clinical features of myelopathy (negative Hoffman and Romberg tests) with normal upper limb tone and reflex testing.

A cervical spinal MRI scan booked by his GP is made available for review (Figure 16.1).

Q: What is the diagnosis?

This patient has a severe right C7–T1 foraminal stenosis and mild flattening of the left ventral cord (mild central canal stenosis) caused by a disc protrusion. Given the absence of CSF effacement and the lack of clinical symptoms of myelopathy, this would not be the primary focus at this stage.

This represents a diagnosis of cervical radiculopathy.

Cervical radiculopathy can be defined as pain, weakness and sensory disturbance in a radicular pattern in one or both upper extremities related to compression and/or irritation of one or more cervical nerve roots. Risk factors include cigarette smoking and prior lumbar radiculopathy.

Q: What other imaging would you request?

I would request an AP and lateral (flexion and extension) plain radiograph of the cervical spine to exclude angular or translational instability.

(a) 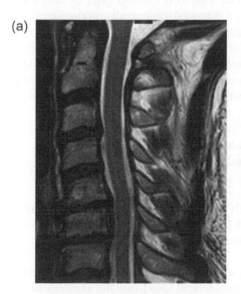 (b)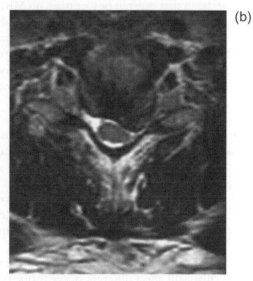

Figure 16.1   MRI scan cervical spine (T2-weighted) (a) sagittal and (b) axial (C7/T1) showing right C7/T1 foraminal stenosis.

DOI: 10.1201/9781003201304-18

(a)

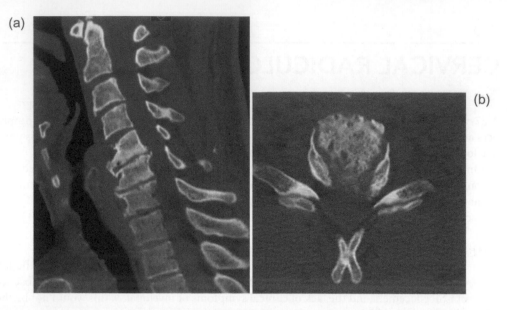

(b)

Figure 16.2 CT scan cervical spine (a) sagittal and (b) axial (C7/T1) showing multilevel degenerative change and right C7/T1 osseous foraminal narrowing.

I would also request a CT scan (Figure 16.2) of the cervical spine to assess whether the protruding disc was calcified as well as to identify the presence of other compressive pathology such as large posterior osteophytes or an OPLL. Identification of large anterior osteophytes and irregularities of the vertebral endplates can also be useful in operative planning.

Computed tomography myelography is indicated for the evaluation of patients with clinical symptoms or signs that are discordant with MRI findings (e.g., foraminal compression that may not be identified on MRI). Computed tomography myelography is also suggested in patients who have a contraindication to MRI.

Electromyography (EMG) is used in many centres as an adjunct to other forms of investigation, but recent evidence-based guideline published in the *Spine Journal* (2020) found insufficient evidence to make a recommendation for or against the use of electromyography for patients in whom the diagnosis of cervical radiculopathy was unclear after clinical examination and MRI.

Q: What are the distinctions between the anatomy of neural structures exiting the cervical spine when compared with the lumbar spine?

The key differences follow:

1. Pedicle/nerve root mismatch

    The cervical spine C6 nerve root travels above the C6 pedicle (*mismatch*), while the lumbar spine L5 nerve root travels under L5 pedicle (*match*). The extra C8 nerve root (no C8 vertebra/pedicle) allows transition to occur.

2. Nerve root orientation

    The orientation of the lumbar nerve roots means that a paracentral and foraminal disc will affect different nerve roots. A paracentral L5/S1 disc herniation will affect the traversing S1 nerve root, while a foraminal disc will affect the exiting L5 nerve root.

Because of the horizontal anatomy of cervical nerve root, a central and foraminal disc will affect the same nerve root; that is, a C7/T1 central or foraminal disc will both affect the C8 nerve root.

3. Nerve roots in the cervical spine take a ventrolateral course from the spinal cord. This predisposes them to ventral compression.

Q: How do causes of foraminal stenosis differ in the cervical, compared to the lumbar, spine?

The most common cause of cervical radiculopathy (in 70–75% of cases) is foraminal encroachment of the spinal nerve due to a combination of factors, including decreased disc height and degenerative changes (i.e., cervical spondylosis; Figure 16.3). In contrast to disorders of the lumbar spine, herniation of the nucleus pulposus is responsible for only 20–25% of cases.

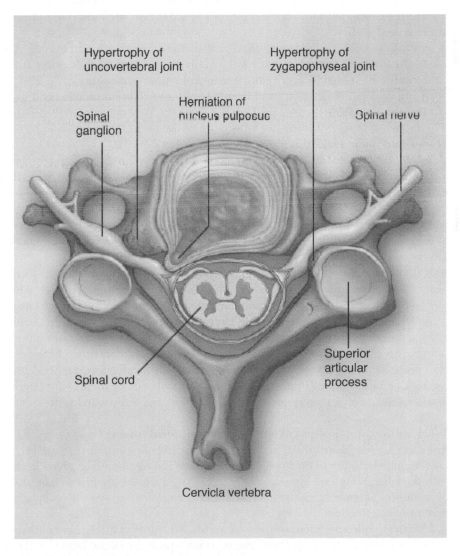

Figure 16.3 Causes of cervical nerve root compression.

Q: What are the most appropriate outcome measures to evaluate the treatment of cervical radiculopathy from degenerative disorders?

The Neck Disability Index, Short Form-36 and Short Form-12, and visual analogue scale are recommended outcome measures for assessing treatments of cervical radiculopathy from degenerative disorders.

Q: What are the anatomical findings of nerve compression at each level of the cervical spine?

- C4: scapular winging, numbness, and pain at the base of the neck
- C5 radiculopathy: deltoid and biceps weakness, diminished biceps reflex pain and numbness in the lateral upper arm
- C6 radiculopathy: brachioradialis and wrist extension weakness, diminished brachioradialis reflex and sensory deficit in the radial forearm and radial two digits
- C7 radiculopathy: triceps and wrist flexion weakness, diminished triceps reflex and sensory deficit in the middle finger, most affected nerve root in cervical radiculopathy in several studies
- C8 radiculopathy: weakness to distal phalanx flexion of middle and index finger (difficulty with fine motor function) and paresthesias in ring and little finger (C8 radiculopathy often manifests in a similar manner to ulnar neuropathy)
- T1 radiculopathy intrinsic hand muscle weakness axillary numbness and ipsilateral Horner's syndrome

Q: How would you manage this patient?

Of patients with radiculopathy, 75% improve with non-operative management. Improvement occurs via the resorption of soft discs and decreased inflammation around irritated nerve roots. If the patient failed a trial of non-operative management, I would consider the use of selective diagnostic and therapeutic CT guided nerve root injections. These have been shown to provides long-term relief in 40–70% of cases but do carry a risk of complications including dural puncture, meningitis, epidural abscess and nerve root injury.

If the patient had a successful diagnostic injection, with only short-term therapeutic benefit, I would consider surgical management. The main indication for surgical management is persistent and disabling pain that has failed 3 months of conservative management.

ACDF remains the gold standard in the surgical treatment of cervical radiculopathy and has an extremely high success rate with a single-level disease. In cases of foraminal soft disc herniation causing single-level radiculopathy, decompression of the nerve root via a posterior foraminotomy (either open or minimally invasive) has reported good outcomes. Contraindications to posterior foraminotomy include patients with large central disc herniation, cervical myelopathy, instability, OPLL and those with kyphotic deformity.

Q: What are the complications of anterior cervical spinal surgery?

Risks include pseudoarthrosis, and 1% risk of recurrent laryngeal nerve (RLN) injury. Less commonly, injury to the hypoglossal nerve and the vertebral artery have been noted, with the latter being rare but potentially fatal. Post-operative dysphagia can be a result of prominent anterior hardware after ACDF or iatrogenic injury to the oesophagus after over-zealous retraction.

Horner's syndrome (characterised by ptosis, anhydrosis, miosis, enophthalmos) is caused by injury to the sympathetic chain, which sits on the lateral border of the longus coli muscle at C6.

Late-stage complications include oesophageal perforation secondary to plate loosening/pull-out and adjacent segment disease, which may necessitate revision surgery.

Exam Tips

- When performing provocative tests, such as Spurling's test (exacerbation of symptoms resulting from foraminal narrowing caused by simultaneous extension and rotation to the affected side, lateral bend and vertical compression reproducing symptoms in the ipsilateral arm), remember that these tests can be painful, and you must carefully watch out for any signs of patient discomfort and discontinue any examination that is causing pain to the patient. Causing unnecessary pain in a viva may well be a pass/fail component!
- Remember that radiographic changes often do not correlate with symptoms. Seventy per cent of patients by 70 years of age will have degenerative changes seen on plain X-rays. Treat the patient, not the scan!
- RLN injury is the most common nerve injury from anterior approach to the cervical spine. Remember that the anatomic course of the nerve differs on the right and left sides. Although theoretically the nerve is at greater risk of injury with a right-sided approach, there is no evidence to support a greater incidence of nerve injury with a right-sided approach.

SUGGESTED READINGS

1. Witzmann A, Hejazi N, Krasznai L. Posterior cervical foraminotomy. A follow-up study of 67 surgically treated patients with compressive radiculopathy. Neurosurg Rev. 2000;23:213–17.
2. Anderberg L, Annertz M, Persson L, et al. Transforaminal steroid injections for the treatment of cervical radiculopathy: a prospective and randomised study. Eur Spine J. 2007;16:321–8.
3. Bono C, Ghiselli G, Gilbert T, et al. An evidence-based clinical guideline for the diagnosis and treatment of cervical radiculopathy from degenerative disorders. Spine J. 2011;11(1):64–72.

17

CERVICAL MYELOPATHY

A 71-year-old male presents via the ED with a 1-year history of posterior neck pain, difficulty walking and recurrent falls. He also complains of a burning sensation in his hands and progressive weakess in his upper and lower extremities.

He has experienced difficulty with fine motor tasks, such as doing his buttons. He presents using a walker and with a stooped posture. He has normal urinary and bowel function. His symptoms have significantly worsened over the last month.

Q: How would you examine this patient?

I would perform a complete neurological exam, including assesment of tone, power, reflexes, sensation (to both pinprick and light touch) and coordination in the upper and lower limbs. I would also perform a gait assessment to exclude ataxia. I would test ankle plantar response bilaterally, as an upward plantar reflex (Babinski sign) can be a sign of upper motor neurone pathology. Limb spasticity and sustained clonus at the ankle would also be relevant findings. I would test proporioception at the big toe and perform a rectal examination to confirm intact anal tone.

Other special tests/signs would include the following:

- Romberg's test
- Hoffman's sign (Figure 17.1; snapping patient's middle distal phalanx leads to spontaneous flexion of the distal interphalangeal joint (DIPJ) and proximal interphalangeal joint (PIPJ) on other fingers)
- Finger escape sign (when the patient holds fingers extended and adducted, the small finger spontaneously abducts due to weakness of intrinsic muscle)
- Grip and release test (myelopathic patients may be unable to make a fist and release 20 times in 10s)
- Lhermitte's sign—test is positive where extreme cervical flexion leads to electric shock-like sensations that radiate down the spine and into the extremities.

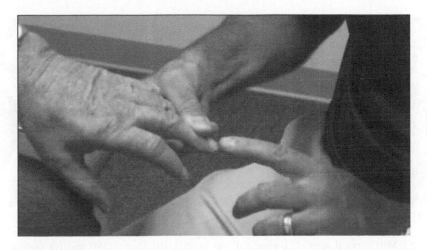

Figure 17.1 Hoffman's sign.

DOI: 10.1201/9781003201304-19

Reflex responses were grade 3 (increased) at the biceps, triceps, brachioradialis, patella and Achilles tendons. Ankle plantar responses were upgoing bilaterally (Babinski sign) with spasticity in the legs and 3 beats of clonus at the ankle. Hoffman's sign was negative. Proprioception testing at the big toe was normal. Sensory examination was normal to light touch. The patient had bilateral weakness in shoulder abduction and elbow flexion, as well as reduced strength of wrist flexion and extension. Digital rectal exam was normal.

Q: What investigations would you perform?

I would initially perform plain radiographs of the cervical spine. I would be specifically looking for osteophyte formation, disc space narrowing and decreased sagittal spinal canal diameter.

I would also look for overall cervical alignment (C2–C7) on a lateral radiograph in the neutral position and would request flexion/extension views to look for angular or translational instability.

An MRI scan of the cervical spine is the gold standard in the investigation of cervical myelopathy. Effacement of CSF indicates functional stenosis. Spinal cord changes (myelomalacia) are seen as a bright signal change on T2 images (Figure 17.2).

Q: What does the MRI scan show?

The MRI shows multilevel degenerative change, with compression of the cervical cord secondary to advanced osteoarthritis of the cervical spine and thickening of the ligamentum flavum. This is consistent with a diagnosis of cervical spondylitic myelopathy (CSM). Cervical stenosis is maximal at the C3/4 level, where there is also cord signal change (myelomalacia). The compression ratio can be calculated from the sagittal view of the MRI scan. (B/A in Figure 17.2c) A compression ratio of less than 0.4 is a poor prognostic indicator.

Q: What investigation would you perform if an MRI scan were contraindicated?

A CT myelogram can be performed in cases in which an MRI scan is contraindicated, such as a pacemaker or due to non-compatible metalwork. However, this is more invasive than an MRI scan and carries a risk of contrast allergy.

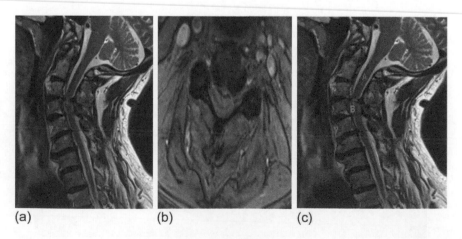

(a)   (b)   (c)

Figure 17.2 MRI cervical spine (T2-weighted) (a) sagittal, (b) axial (C3/4) and (c) sagittal (marked) showing cervical stenosis, maximal a C3/4 with myelomalacia.

Q: Why is urinary dysfunction associated with spinal cord compression in some cases?

Spinal cord injury (SCI) interrupts the brainstem signals coordinating detrusor contraction and sphincter relaxation, leading to 'detrusor-sphincter dyssynergia'. This causes incomplete emptying, urinary urgency and overflow incontinence. SCI should be suspected in patients presenting with urinary dysfunction and limb weakness because innervation of the bladder arises caudal to innervation of the limbs; therefore, if the limbs are affected by SCI, the bladder will likely be affected as well.

Q: How would you definitively manage this patient?

Management of CSM is dependent on the severity and progression of the patient's symptoms, as well as the imaging findings, rather than either of these in isolation. Non-operative management, with observation, analgesia and therapy, can be appropriate in patients with minimal cervical stenosis on MRI scan and mild disease without significant functional impairment.

In this case, operative management is warranted because of the significant stenosis and functional impairment. The aim of surgery is decompression and stabilisation of the compressed region of the spinal cord segment.

A decision on the optimal surgical approach can be helped using a CT scan cervical spine (Figure 17.3). This is better than MRI scan at identifying large osteophytes, disc calcification and ossification of the posterior longitudinal ligament (OPLL; Figure 17.4).

a ACDF is the mainstay of the management of patients with 1 or 2 level compression. It should be performed for functionally impaired patients with cervical stenosis caused by

- compression arising from 2 or fewer disc segments,
- anterior pathology (non-calcified disc, disc osteophyte complexes),
- no involvement of ligamentum flavum in compression of the spinal cord and
- fixed cervical kyphosis of >10 degrees.

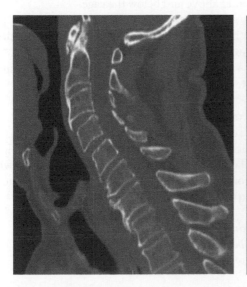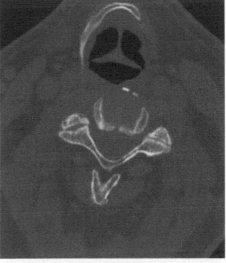

Figure 17.3 CT cervical spine sagittal and axial (C3/4) showing C2/3 ankylosis with a large anterior osteophyte at the anterolateral aspect of the C3 vertebra.

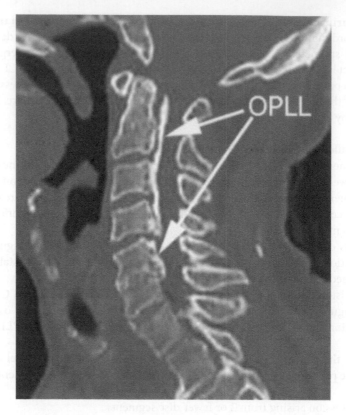

Figure 17.4   Example of OPLL.

Fixation can be achieved by anterior plating or via screws which go through the ACDF cage and fix it to the cervical vertebral bodies above and below the cage.

b Anterior corpectomy and fusion (ACF) should be performed for functionally impaired patients with cervical stenosis caused by extensive retro vertebral disease.
c Posterior decompression (laminectomy) +/− stabilisation should be performed for functionally impaired patients with cervical stenosis caused by

- multilevel compression with kyphosis of <10 degrees and
- >13 degrees of fixed kyphosis which is a contraindication for a posterior procedure. This is because posterior decompression relies on the decompressed spinal cord being able to drift back into the space created by the laminectomy. This cannot occur in a patient with a fixed cervical kyphosis. Posterior decompression can be effective in a flexible kyphotic spine if it can be corrected prior to instrumentation on extension views.

This patient has C3–5 stenosis, with maximal compression at C3/4 from a buckled ligamentum flavum. This would not have been possible to access via an anterior only approach. A posterior laminectomy and fusion were performed to decompress the stenotic segment of the cervical spine (Figure 17.5).

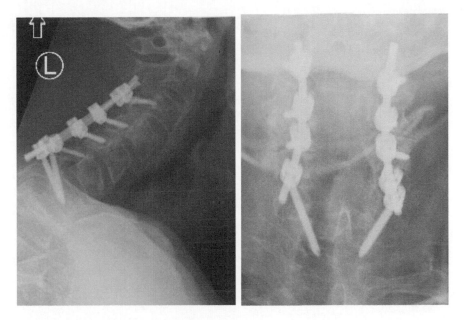

Figure 17.5   Post-operative plain radiograph cervical spine.

Q: How would you consent this patient for this procedure?

Risks of posterior cervical decompression include bleeding (including from injury to the vertebral artery), pseudoarthrosis, postoperative C5 palsy, hardware failure and migration and proximal junctional kyphosis.

Risks of anterior cervical decompression include oesophageal injury, recurrent laryngeal nerve (RLN) injury, C5 palsy and post-operative haematoma.

The aim of surgery is to ***prevent the progression*** of symptoms. Recovery from established SCI is less predictable.

SUGGESTED READINGS

1.   Zhang Y-Z, Shen Y, Wang LF, et al. Magnetic resonance T2 image signal intensity ratio and clinical manifestation predict prognosis after surgical intervention for cervical spondylotic myelopathy. Spine (Phila Pa 1976). 2010;35(10):E396–9.
2.   Yukawa Y, Kato F, Yoshihara H, et al. MR T2 image classification in cervical compression myelopathy: predictor of surgical outcomes. Spine (Phila Pa 1976). 2007;32(15):1675–8.
3.   Bingxuan W, Baoge L, Dacheng S, et al. The association between cervical focal kyphosis and myelopathy severity in patients with cervical spondylotic myelopathy before surgery. Eur Spine J. 2021;30(6):1501–8.

18

THORACIC DISC

You are called to see a 54-year-old woman with a 6-week history of worsening midline back pain and numbness circumferentially around her rib cage. She also complains of intermittent bilateral leg weakness and numbness. She denies bowel or bladder changes.

On examination, she has Medical Research Council (MRC) grade 4 power on hip, knee and ankle flexion/extension. She was hyper-reflexic on the patella tendon and ankle-jerk testing, with 3 beats of clonus bilaterally. She has a positive Romberg test and a broad-based ataxic gait. She has patchy sensory changes in the lower limbs without a defined dermatomal distribution. Rectal examination and perianal sensation are normal.

She has been seen by her General Practitioner (GP) 2 weeks previously, who requested an outpatient X-ray and MRI scan (Figure 18.1) but presents emergently due to an acute worsening of her lower limb weakness and back pain.

Q: What is the diagnosis?

This patient has central thoracic stenosis at the T11–T12 level caused by the disc osteophyte complex. There is also a focal area of myelomalacia (cord signal change).

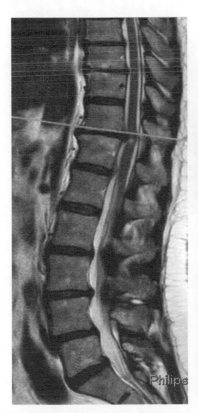
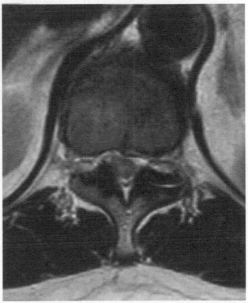

Figure 18.1   MRI scan (T2-weighted) thoracolumbar spine showing thoracic (T11/12) stenosis.

DOI: 10.1201/9781003201304-20

In 75% of cases, the disc herniation is located below the T7–T8 disc. Only 4% of TDHs are located above T3–T4. The T11–T12 disc is the most vulnerable because of greater mobility and posterior longitudinal ligament weakness at this level. TDHs are more common in adults 30–50 years of age. Cases of TDH complicating proximal junctional syndrome after thoracolumbar fusion have been reported.

Q: How can TDH be classified?

TDH can either be classified by the location of the herniation or the herniation type.

Herniation can be described as central, posterolateral, lateral (location classification) or can be described as bulging (nucleus annulus remains intact), extruded (disc pushes through annulus but confined by PLL) or sequestered (disc material free in canal).

Q: Would you request any other imaging?

TDH is frequently associated with ossification of the thoracic disc or the ligamentum flavum (OLF). In rare cases, calcified herniations are an extension of the nucleus pulposus, which is itself calcified. A giant TDH is one that occupies more than 40% of the spinal canal, and giant calcified TDHs have an intradural extension in 15–70% of cases.

A CT scan (Figure 18.2) of the thoracic spine would help identify calcification/ossification more clearly than a plain radiograph.

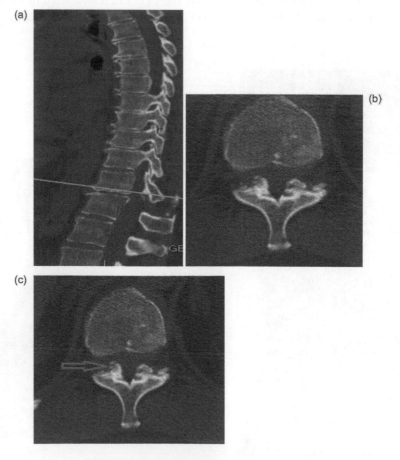

Figure 18.2 CT scan showing ossification of the ligamentum flavum at the affected level (T11/12) marked in (c). a–c : (clockwise) (a) sagittal view CT scan thoracic spine (b) axial view CT scan (T11/12 level) (c) axial view.

Q: What are the common presentations of this condition?

The main clinical sign is pain, which is present in 92% of cases (intercostal neuralgia, back pain). Neurological deficits can be either sensory or motor in the context of slow medullary compression, while ataxia during walking or progressive deficits of the lower limbs are also common. Giant calcified TDHs are discovered because of myelopathy in 70–95% of cases. Myelopathy is present in only 47% of cases of non-calcified TDHs.

Q: Why is the thoracic cord particularly vulnerable to compression?

- Thoracic kyphosis flattens the dural sheath against the posterior portion of the disc and the denticulate ligaments limit the spinal cord's mobility within the dural sheath, making it more vulnerable.
- The diameter of the spinal cord (6.5 × 8 mm) is large relative to the diameter of the thoracic spinal canal (16.8 × 17.2 mm), which leaves little free space around the spinal cord.
- There is an area of poor thoracic medullary vascularisation called the "watershed zone".

Q: How would you manage this patient?

Most cases can be managed non-operatively with a combination of **activity modification, physical therapy, oral analgesia and** therapeutic nerve root injections for well-defined radiculopathic pain. Surgery is indicated in patients with functional symptoms that do not respond to medical treatment and/or those with neurological symptoms. The presence of signs of cord compression on MRI scan (intramedullary hypointense T1 signal and hyperintense T2 signal)—even in the absence of neurological symptoms—can be a surgical indication.

There is considerable debate over whether anterior or posterior approaches are optimal and whether fusion is needed in all cases.

Surgical approaches include the following:

- **Anterior approaches** such as the transpleural thoracotomy, thoracoscopy (which can be done via video-assisted thoracic surgery [VATS]) and mini-thoracotomy with retropleural variation
- **Posterolateral approaches** such as the transpedicular discectomy or/and trans-facet variations that spare the pedicle
- **Lateral approaches** such as the costo-transversectomy (the removal of a section of the medial rib and rib head, plus transverse process to access a lateral disc herniation)

The optimal approach depends on the consistency of the herniation and its location related to the spinal cord. Centrally located large, calcified discs can be approached via anterior or lateral approaches, whereas non-calcified or lateral herniated discs can be treated from anterior, lateral or posterior approaches. Posterior approaches almost always require instrumented fusion.

The use of intraoperative neuro-monitoring is commonly described for these procedures. Pre-operative arteriography, to locate the Adamkiewicz artery (the dominant thoracolumbar segmental artery that supplies the spinal cord) can also be useful to decide the preferred side of a transthoracic approach.

One major complication in the thoracic spine is wrong level surgery. This is a 'never event'. Care should be taken to identify the correct level pre-operatively once in the OR. Various techniques include K-wire inserted into the pedicle during the surgery under fluoroscopic control or a micro-puncture needle used to leave a marker on the periosteum of the pedicle.

Exam Tips

- Identification of calcification of a thoracic disc and/or of the ligamentum flavum is key, and so CT scans are essential, but MRI scans are the gold standard of investigation.
- Always remember to examine the patients' upper limbs, as some patients will have tandem thoracic and cervical stenosis. A whole-spine MRI is useful to exclude this.

SUGGESTED READINGS

1. Arts MP, Bartels RH. Anterior or posterior approach of thoracic disc herniation? A comparative cohort of mini-transthoracic versus transpedicular discectomies. Spine J. 2014;14(8):1654–62.
2. Court C, Mansour E, Bouthors C. Thoracic disc herniation: surgical treatment. Orthop Traumatol Surg Res. 2018;104(1S):S31–S40.
3. Paolini S, Tola S, Missori P, et al. Endoscope-assisted resection of calcified thoracic disc herniations. Eur Spine J. 2016;25(1):200–6.

19

LUMBAR STENOSIS

You are referred a 53-year-old man from his general practitioner (GP), with a 6-month history of lumbar spinal and left-sided leg pain with radiation into the lateral calf. He has difficulty walking upstairs because his left foot 'catches' against the step above as he climbs. He denies any bowel or bladder dysfunction. He has had no recent weight loss or other red-flag signs.

He is a retired plumber and has no other medical history. He had spent 3 months in intensive physiotherapy without improvement of symptoms. An outpatient MRI scan lumbar spine is provided (Figure 19.1).

Q: What is the diagnosis?

This patient has disc degeneration at the L4/5 level with modic endplate changes. There is a left-sided paracentral disc protrusion causing central stenosis, with compression of the traversing L5 nerve root.

Q: How would you examine this patient?

I would perform a focused examination. This would include assessment of tone, power, reflexes, sensation and coordination in the lower and upper limbs. Specifically, I would expect the plantar reflexes to be downward, as this pathology is a lower motor neurone lesion. I would examine lower limb power with a particular focus on any weakness in the L5 myotome (great toe dorsiflexion), and I would examine for light touch and pinprick sensation throughout the left leg compared to the contralateral side, focusing on the L5 dermatome. Any abnormalities in the neurological examination of the upper limbs or any

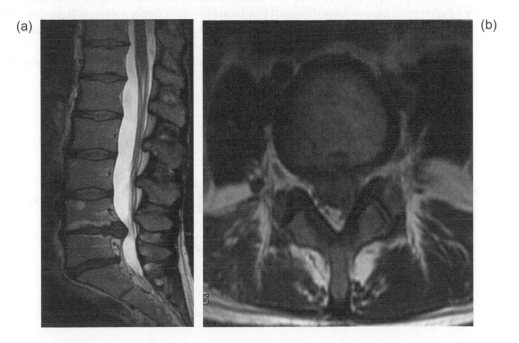

(a)   (b)

Figure 19.1   MRI scan (T2-weighted) lumbar spine (a) sagittal and (b) axial (L4/5).

DOI: 10.1201/9781003201304-21

signs of an upper motor neurone lesion, (such as hypertonia, clonus, hyperreflexia or an upgoing plantar reflex) would make me consider the possibility of 'tandem' cervical stenosis. If this were present, I would request an MRI scan of the cervical and thoracic spine before considering any further management of the lumbar spine.

Finally, I would perform provocative 'special' tests. These include the straight leg raise (SLR) (done with the patient supine or sitting), which if positive would lead to the reproduction of pain and paraesthesia in the affected area at 30–70 degrees of flexion. Lesegue's sign is the aggravation of symptoms on SLR with ankle dorsiflexion.

I would finally perform a gait analysis. A broad-based gait or ataxia can be a sign of tandem cervical or thoracic stenosis, a foot drop can be caused by a weakness in ankle dorsiflexion (L4), while a Trendelenburg gait can be caused by a gluteus medius weakness (L5).

Q: How can disc protrusion be classified?
Classification can be anatomical or by location.

Anatomical:

- Protrusion (eccentric bulge with intact annulus fibrosis)
- Extrusion (herniation of disc material through annulus fibrosis which remains within the disc space)
- Sequestered fragment (free)—herniated disc material no longer continuous with disc space.

Classification by location is relevant in terms of which spinal nerve root is compressed by the disc (Figure 19.2):

- Central prolapse (may present with cauda equina syndrome—surgical emergency)
- Paracentral (posterolateral)—most common (90–95%) due to a disc prolapse through the weakest part of the PLL. Affects the traversing nerve root, that is, L4/5 paracentral disc affects the traversing L5 nerve root
- Foraminal/far lateral—less common (5–10%) affects the exiting nerve root, that is, L4/5 far lateral disc affects the exiting L4 nerve root

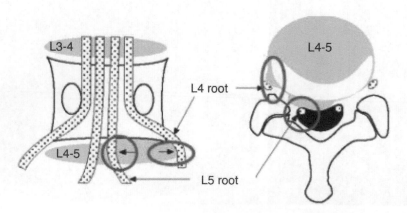

Figure 19.2 Organisation of the exiting and traversing nerve roots in the Lumbar spine.

Q: How would you manage this patient?

This patient should be managed in a stepwise approach.

The first line of treatment is non-operative management—rest, physiotherapy, and anti-inflammatory medications. Of patients with disc herniation, 90% can be successfully managed without surgery. A significant proportion of acute herniation undergoes spontaneous resorption as the disc becomes dehydrated, reducing pressure on the affected nerve root.

The second line of treatment is via X-ray or CT-guided corticosteroid and local anaesthetic injections. These can be both diagnostic and therapeutic. A significant improvement in symptoms is an indication that the pain generator has been identified, even if the improvement if short-lived. Caudal epidural injections do not target a particular nerve root but can lead to significant pain relief. Injections lead to improvement in around 50% of patients at 6 months.

The third line of treatment is via operative management (laminectomy and microdiscectomy).

Indications for surgical management are

- persistent disabling pain >6 weeks that has failed conservative treatment,
- progressive and significant weakness and
- cauda equina syndrome.

This can be performed via open, mini-open or minimally invasive (tubular or endoscopic) approaches through the midline for central and paracentral discs, while a paraspinal (Wiltse) approach can be used for far lateral discs.

Q: What are the possible complications of decompressive surgery?

The major risks of laminectomy and microdiscectomy include dural tear (1%), recurrent disc prolapse, and discitis (1%). There is also a risk of secondary instability if too much of the facet joint (generally thought to be about 50%) is removed during the laminectomy.

Q: What are the indications for fusion in addition to decompression?

One of the major controversies about surgery for spinal stenosis is the role of spinal fusion. Fusion has generally been recommended for spinal stenosis associated with degenerative unstable spondylolisthesis.

While this is a controversial area, there are some recommendations from the World Federation of Neurosurgical Societies:

- In patients with lumbar spine stenosis and no sign or symptoms of instability and predominant leg pain, decompression alone is recommended.
- In patients with stenosis and stable spondylolisthesis, fusion is not mandatory, and decompression alone is suggested.
- Unstable spondylolisthesis with symptoms may require fusion.
- Fusion may be advisable in patients who undergo bilateral facetectomy of more than 50% and bilateral discectomy.
- There is no consensus if the main complaint is mechanical axial low back pain, which is more than leg pain; the patient may benefit from a fusion surgery.

Guidelines from the North American Spine Society (NASS) recommend that in the absence of associated scoliosis or spondylolisthesis, 'decompression alone is suggested for patients with predominant leg symptoms without instability'. Instability can be assessed by flexion and extension views of the lumbar spine.

Exam Tips

- This is a frequently tested subject. An awareness of the relevant myotomes and dermatomes related to the entire spine (especially cervical and lumbar) is essential. You should make sure you fully understand the association between the location of the disc prolapse and the affected nerve root.
- Different spinal surgeons have conflicting views on the role of fusion surgery versus discectomy/decompression alone. An awareness of the existence of controversy and some awareness of the evidence on either side should be sufficient to score well here.
- Of patients with lumbar stenosis, 50% will have some degree of so-called tandem cervical stenosis. Keep this in mind and order further imaging if there is any clinical suspicion of spinal cord involvement.

SUGGESTED READINGS

1. Lurie J, Tomkins-Lane C. Management of lumbar spinal stenosis. BMJ. 2016;352:h6234.
2. Zaina F, Tomkins-Lane C, Carragee E, et al. Surgical versus non-surgical treatment for lumbar spinal stenosis. Cochrane Database Syst Rev. 2016;2016(1):CD010264.
3. Shen J, Xu S, Xu S, et al. Fusion or not for degenerative lumbar spinal stenosis: a meta-analysis and systematic review. Pain Physician. 2018;21(1):1–8.

20

LUMBAR STENOSIS WITH ACHONDROPLASIA

A 32-year-old lady with achondroplasia presents with a 6-month history of bilateral shooting posterior leg pain, weakness and heaviness after a walking distance of around 150 yards, denies bowel or bladder symptoms.

She underwent a posterior cervical decompression for cervical stenosis 5 years previously.

On examination, she is of short stature with normal trunk height and characteristic physical features of achondroplasia, including frontal bossing.

Q: What investigation would you perform?

I would perform an AP and lateral (Figure 20.1) plain radiograph of the whole spine, as well as MRI scans (Figure 20.2) of the whole spine. Patients with achondroplasia have an increased incidence of lumbar and foramen magnum stenosis, as well as spinal deformities such as lumbar hyperlordosis and thoracolumbar kyphosis. The whole spine should be fully radiographically investigated to obtain a complete diagnosis.

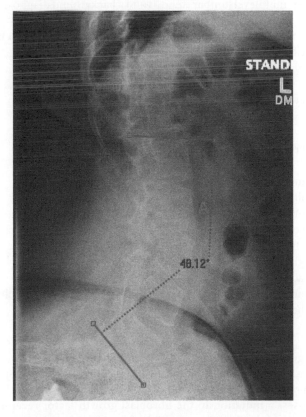

Figure 20.1 X-ray lumbar spine (lateral) showing lumbo-sacral lordosis of 48 degrees in a patient with achondroplasia.

DOI: 10.1201/9781003201304-22

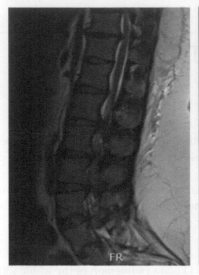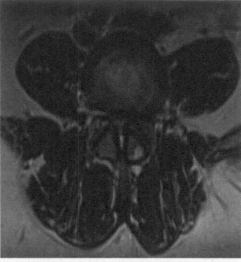

Figure 20.2 MRI scan (T2-weighted) lumbar spine sagittal and axial (L4/5) showing multilevel lumbar stenosis.

Q: What is the diagnosis?

This patient has multilevel lumbar stenosis and a background diagnosis of achondroplasia.

Q: What are the other classical orthopaedic findings on examination of patients with achondroplasia?

Lumbar spinal findings include

- vertebral wedging in thoracolumbar kyphosis and
- posterior vertebral scalloping.

Pelvis and extremity findings include

- champagne glass pelvis (pelvis width >depth),
- squared iliac wings,
- 'inverted V' shape of distal femoral physis,
- rhizomelic dwarfism (humerus shorter than forearm and femur shorter than tibia and a normal trunk),
- adult height ~50 inches,
- radial head subluxation,
- trident hands (fingers same length with divergent ring and middle fingers) and
- genu varum.

Q: What is the genetic background of achondroplasia?

Achondroplasia is the most common form of human skeletal dysplasia, with an estimated frequency of between 1 in 15,000 and 1 in 40,000 live births. Patients with achondroplasia possess a mutation in the fibroblast growth factor receptor-3 (FGFR3) gene on the short arm of chromosome 4, which affects the maturation of chondrocytes in the growth plate.

The transmission of achondroplasia is by an autosomal dominant inheritance, although 80–90% of patients have additional new mutations.

Q: How should this patient be managed?

Non-operative management (weight loss, physical therapy, corticosteroid injections) is indicated in mild to moderate lumbar stenosis as first-line treatment. Surgical management (multilevel laminectomy ± fusion) is indicated in spinal stenosis with severe symptoms or where nonoperative management has failed.

Care should be taken of the anatomical abnormalities that may make surgery more challenging in achondroplasia. These include thoracic hyper-kyphosis and the patient's short stature which may make patient positioning more challenging, as well as shortened pedicles and decreased interpedicular distance, which should be taken into consideration at pre-operative planning.

Exam Tip

- Achondroplasia is a rare diagnosis and therefore less likely to be faced in an FRCS viva scenario than other more common conditions. The key when faced when a rare scenario when you know that more challenging questions may be coming (e.g., genetic inheritance) is to go back to basics and pick up marks where possible. Identifying and talking in more general terms about lumbar stenosis, with an awareness of the fact that you should investigate the cervical spine and mentioning the possible difficulties of positioning the patient due to their stature are examples of how this can be done effectively.

SUGGESTED READINGS

1. Thomeer RT, van Dijk JM. Surgical treatment of lumbar stenosis in achondroplasia. J Neurosurg. 2002;96:292–7.
2. Srikumaran U, et al. Pedicle and spinal canal parameters of the lower thoracic and lumbar vertebrae in the achondroplast population. Spine. 2007;32(22):2423–31.

21

SYNOVIAL CYST

You are referred a 68-year-old retired labourer who presents with a 7-month history of severe right-sided leg pain with radiation into his calf and lateral aspect of his right foot.

On examination, he has normal motor and sensory function in both legs, except for slight weakness in right great toe extension (Medical Research Council (MRC) grade 3). He had completed 6 months of non-operative management with rest, physiotherapy and NSAIDs. He has no bowel or bladder symptoms.

An outpatient MRI scan of the lumbar spine has been requested by his general practitioner. (Figure 21.1)

Q: What is the diagnosis?

There is an extradural lesion at the L4/5 level causing paracentral lumbar stenosis and compressing the traversing L5 nerve root. This radiologically appears to be a synovial facet cyst. These are degenerative lesions found most commonly at the L4/5 level (most mobile segment). They are classically associated with mechanical back pain and/or radicular symptoms.

Q: What other images would you request?

There is some evidence that that synovial cyst herniation might be a manifestation of an unstable spinal level.

I would request flexion and extension views of the lumbar spine to exclude segmental instability/dynamic spondylolisthesis. If there was evidence of instability, I would consider fusion rather than decompression alone.

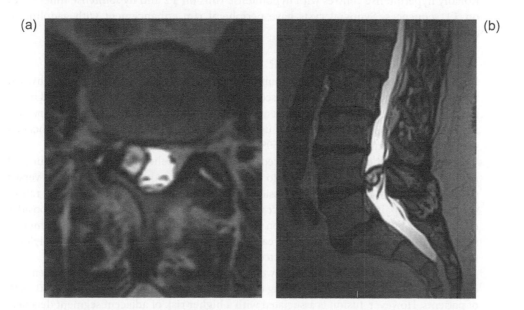

Figure 21.1   MRI scan (T2-weighted) (a) lumbar spine showing (b) right-sided L4/5 synovial cyst.

DOI: 10.1201/9781003201304-23

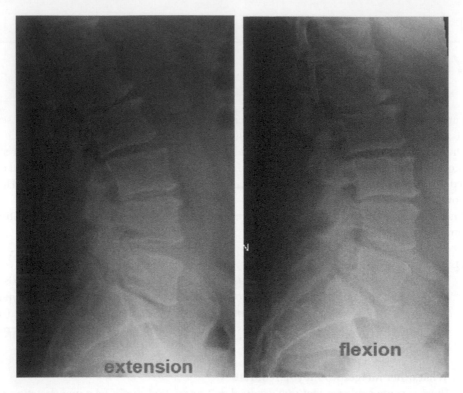

Figure 21.2   Flexion and extension lumbar spinal X-rays showing grade 1 spondylolisthesis (<25%) L5/S1.

If there was significant query about the diagnosis after the initial MRI scan, I would consider an MRI scan with gadolinum enhancement. Synovial cysts on MRI scans traditionally hyperintense centres with hypointense rims on T2 and hypointense inner cores on T1 sequences. Synovial cysts have peripheral rim enhancement with gadolinium contrast.

Q: How should this patient be managed?
In a patient who had completed 6 months of conservative management with physical therapy, I would consider CT or fluoroscopically guided cyst rupture ± facet steroid injection. This is the second line management of patients who have failed initial conservative management. It has pain relief rates of up to 75% at 1 year, but it is reportedly associated with secondary surgery rates of up to 50%.

If this failed or the patient experienced only short-term relief, I would consider surgical management. This is some debate as to the indications for decompression alone versus decompression and fusion. Decompression alone has been associated with a higher rate of recurrent back pain and cyst recurrence in some studies, while many specialists consider dynamic instability on flexion/extension view to be an absolute indication for decompression and fusion. Decompression alone carries an increased risk of iatrogenic spondylolisthesis if >50% of the facet joint is resected.

Facetectomy and fusion have the lowest risk of persistent back pain and recurrence of cyst formation in recent studies, leading to a complete resolution of symptoms in 80–90% of patients. However, fusion is associated with a higher risk of adjacent segment degeneration compared with decompression alone.

One specific risk of decompression surgery in the presence of a synovial cyst (with or without fusion) is dural tear. This is due to the risk of adherence of the synovial cyst to the dural sac.

SUGGESTED READINGS

1. Ramhmdani S, Ishida W, Perdomo-Pantoja A, et al. Synovial cyst as a marker for lumbar instability: a systematic review and meta-analysis. World Neurosurg. 2019;122:e1059–68.
2. Wun K, Hashmi SZ, Maslak J, et al. The variability of lumbar facet joint synovial cyst recurrence requiring revision surgery after decompression-only and decompression/fusion. Clin Spine Surg. 2019;32(10):F457–61.
3. Khan AM, Girardi F. Spinal lumbar synovial cysts. Diagnosis and management challenge. Eur Spine J. 2006;15(8):1176–82.

22

CAUDA EQUINA SYNDROME

A 42-year-old lady is referred to the orthopaedic on-call team from the ED with a 9h history of worsening back pain, leg weakness, bilateral leg pain and 2 episodes of urinary incontinence. She has no history of previous spinal surgery and has two children aged 5 and 7, both delivered by vaginal delivery without significant complications.

An X-ray lumbar spine and MRI lumbar spine (Figure 22.1) was performed.

Q: What is the diagnosis, and how would this be confirmed?

The working diagnosis in this case would be cauda equina syndrome (CES) secondary to an L4/5 disc prolapse. This is a surgical emergency with the potential for significant morbidity and long-term neurologic deficits. Risk factors include obesity and female gender. Large central disc herniation or prolapse at the L4/L5 or L5/S1 level accounts for over 45% of cases. While disc herniation is the most common cause of CES, only 1–2% of all disc herniations will result in CES.

I would take a thorough history, particularly focused on the duration of symptoms and the nature of the urinary incontinence (urge vs overflow). The physical examination may be challenging in these patients, particularly if they are in severe pain. Therefore, I would administer suitable analgesia to ensure that a reliable examination could be performed. My examination would focus on assessing power and sensation of the lower extremities (L2–S3), perianal region sensation (S2–S4), patellar reflex (L4), the Achilles tendon reflex (S1), anal wink reflex (assessed by gently stroking the skin around the anus with a cotton swab or applicator—an intact reflex results in contraction of the external anal sphincter) and the bulbocavernosus reflex (S2–4; anal sphincter contraction in response to squeezing the glans penis or pulling on a urinary catheter).

(a) 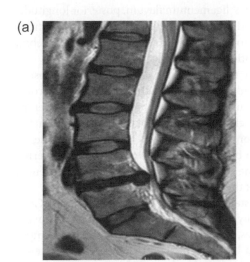 (b)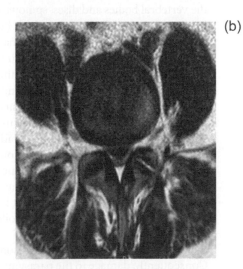

Figure 22.1 MRI scans (a) sagittal and (b) axial (L4/5) lumbar spine.

DOI: 10.1201/9781003201304-24

The Achilles and patellar reflexes are typically reduced in CES, but hyperreflexia may be present when the compression is multifocal or superior to the cauda equina. An absent anal wink reflex is associated with dysfunction of the sacral nerve roots. This is typically absent in CES. While a rectal examination is still recommended as part of the complete examination of possible CES, the literature suggests rectal tone findings are not well correlated with CES.

A post void ultrasound bladder scan should also be performed as part of the diagnostic pathway. A 2009 study by Domen et al. found that a post-void volume >500mL had an odds ratio of 4.0 for diagnosing CES. However, the odds ratio increased to 48.0 when this was combined with two of the following three symptoms: bilateral sciatica, subjective complaints of urinary retention or rectal incontinence symptoms.

Q: What are the relevant clinical features of CES?

While back pain is the most common symptom in CES, other symptoms include unilateral or bilateral sciatica, decreased perianal region sensation, faecal and bladder disruption, lower extremity weakness and reduced sexual function. However, many patients do not present with all these symptoms, and they may occur either suddenly or gradually. Retention typically precedes incontinence; therefore, patients may not present with incontinence until late in the disease process.

Some authors have categorised CES further into CES incomplete (CESI) and CES complete with urinary retention (CESR). CESR describes painless urinary retention with overflow incontinence and complete perianal sensory loss. CESI symptoms include loss of desire to void, altered urinary sensation, and hesitancy with partial saddle anaesthesia. The presence of saddle anaesthesia or bladder dysfunction is associated with worse outcomes.

Describe the relevant anatomy of this condition. (Figure 22.2)

The spinal cord ends with the conus medullaris at the L1/L2 vertebral level, which then travels further as nerve roots. These nerve roots include the ascending and descending nerve roots from L2 through the coccygeal segments. These nerves control lower limb movement (L2–S2), lower limb sensation (L2–S3), bladder control (S2–S4), external anal sphincter control (S2–S4), external genitalia and perianal sensation (S2–S4) and coccygeal sensation (S4, S5, and the coccygeal nerve).

The nerve roots travel within the vertebral canal and are surrounded by the neural arches, the vertebral bodies and discs, spinous processes, ligamentum flavum, posterior longitudinal ligaments and facet joints, which house and protect the nerve roots. CES results from any compression of these cauda equina nerve roots along their course within the vertebral canal, including direct compression, inflammation, venous congestion or ischemia.

The bladder's innervation is via the pelvic splanchnic nerves (S2–S4), with sensory input from the hypogastric, pelvic and pudendal nerves, while the autonomic control is primarily via the parasympathetic system. Stimulation of these nerves causes bladder emptying through stimulation of the detrusor muscle and inhibition of the urethral sphincter. Damage to these nerves results in bladder atony with urinary retention and the absence of voluntary control. Defecation is controlled by the internal (involuntary) and external (voluntary) anal sphincters. Stimulation of the rectum from stool triggers the pudendal nerve (S2–S4) to increase peristalsis and relax the sphincters.

Damage to these nerves can result in aperistalsis and failure of sphincter activity. Constipation is generally the first sign, followed by failure to voluntarily retain stool. Sexual function can also be affected by CES. In males, erection is controlled by the parasympathetic system, while ejaculation is controlled by the sympathetic and somatic systems. Consequently, damage to the parasympathetic innervation from CES will result in erectile dysfunction.

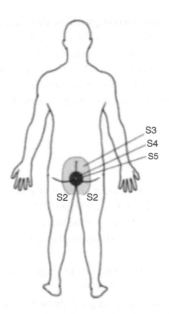

Illustration of saddle anesthesia;
- The S5, S4, and S3 nerves provide sensory innervation to the rectum, perineum, and inner thigh.

Figure 22.2   Dermatomal illustration of saddle anaesthesia.

Q: What is the investigation of choice if an MRI scan is contraindicated?

When MRI cannot be performed, clinicians should consider a CT myelogram. CT myelography is more invasive than MRI and involves placing a needle into the spinal canal followed by injection of contrast dye.

Q: How should this patient be definitively managed?

Treatment involves immediate spinal consultation for surgical decompression. The literature suggests that surgery should be performed within 48 h of symptoms with abrupt onset, as delays beyond 48 h are associated with a greater risk of permanent dysfunction. While the exact timing for surgical management is controversial, those with rapid onset of symptoms (defined as occurring within 24h) or evolving bladder dysfunction are considered particularly high risk, and several studies recommend that these patients undergo surgery within 24h of presentation.

Q: What is the evidence on the timing of surgery?

The evidence on the timing of surgery is mixed. Srikandarajah et al. retrospectively analysed the effect of early (<24h) decompression, finding a lower rate of bladder dysfunction in CESI patients at initial follow-up in patients who underwent early decompression. Heyes et al. retrospectively reviewed 136 patients treated with CES, finding no association between early (<24h) decompression surgery and significantly improved outcomes of bowel or bladder dysfunction, compared with those patients who underwent delayed decompression.

Exam Tip

• Cauda equina is a surgical emergency and therefore is frequently tested. To score well here, you should have a couple of ready to quote references concerning the timing of surgery and diagnosis. Candidates often get very hung up on the question regarding timing of surgery. The literature is mixed. In essence, decompression should be performed as soon as safely possible. Decompression within 24h is the safest answer to the timing question. From our experience, patients admitted overnight (after midnight) can be booked for first thing on a morning emergency list rather than operated on overnight. This recognises literature suggesting that operative outcomes are less good when surgeons are tired and there is a lack of medical and anaesthetic support.

SUGGESTED READINGS

1. Domen PM, Hofman PA, van Santbrink H, et al. Predictive value of clinical characteristics in patients with suspected cauda equina syndrome. Eur J Neurol. 2009;16(3):416–19.
2. Korse NS, Pijpers JA, van Zwet E, et al. Cauda equina syndrome: presentation, outcome, and predictors with focus on micturition, defecation, and sexual dysfunction. Eur Spine J. 2017;26(3):894–904.
3. Todd NV. Guidelines for cauda equina syndrome. Red flags and white flags. Systematic review and implications for triage. Br J Neurosurg. 2017;31(3):336–9.
4. Srikandarajah N, Boissaud-Cooke M, Clark S, et al. Does early surgical decompression in cauda equina syndrome improve bladder outcome? Spine. 2015;40(8):580–3.
5. Heyes G, Jones M, Verzin E, et al. Influence of timing of surgery on Cauda equina syndrome: outcomes at a national spinal centre. J Orthop. 2018;15(1):210–15.

23

ADULT DEGENERATIVE SPONDYLOLISTHESIS

Q: A 70-year-old male presents to your clinic with a 4-year history of worsening lower back pain and bilateral buttock and lower extremity pain. He has no bladder or bowel dysfunction. Walking distance is 20 steps prior to the onset of symptoms. Repeated epidural steroid injections have now become ineffective. Examination reveals he stands with a flexed posture, a normal neurological examination and a normal vascular examination. His upright X-ray (XR) and MRI is as shown. Can you comment on the imaging and suggest the cause for his symptoms?

This is an upright XR of the lumbar spine showing a spondylolisthesis at the L4/5 level. According to the Meyerding classification, this would be a grade 1 spondylolisthesis. The most likely diagnosis in a patient of this age and at the L4/5 level is a degenerate spondylolisthesis. Disc degeneration leads to micromotion of the entire segment. The facet capsules stretch and degenerate which leads to macromotion, and eventual listhesis. The slip becomes more pronounced when weight-bearing as demonstrated. The slip causes central and lateral recess stenosis. This is augmented by the degenerate hypertrophied facets as well as hypertrophied ligamentum. The traversing L5 nerve roots are affected in the lateral recess and the sacral nerve roots in the central canal.

This effect is augmented on weight-bearing and is likely to be responsible for this patient's symptoms, which is why the walking distance is now so limited. Foraminal stenosis may also occur because of disc degeneration and collapse, facet arthrosis and osteophytes from the vertebral body. These features are all demonstrated on this patient's MRI including the presence of facet effusions indicating instability.

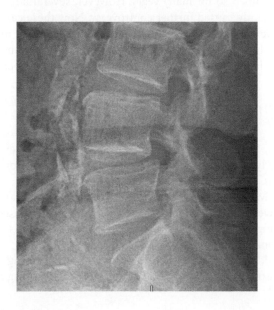

DOI: 10.1201/9781003201304-25

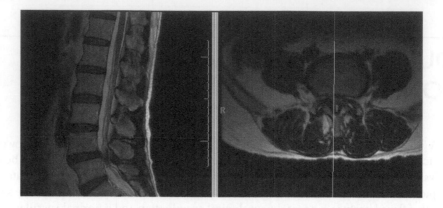

Q: What are the treatment options available for this patient?

This patient has central stenosis and needs this to be addressed with a laminectomy via a midline approach. However, he may also require fusion either with posterior instrumentation or the addition of an interbody cage. I would like to review the MRI scan more comprehensively to assess the neural foramen. If a significant degree of foraminal stenosis exists, then this needs to be addressed either via direct or indirect decompression. Direct decompression by resecting the facets and inserting a transforaminal lumbar interbody fusion (TLIF) cage on the most affected side would address this problem and lend stability via fusion. Using an anterior lumbar interbody fusion (ALIF) cage to effect indirect decompression for this purpose may be used but is far less common in degenerate spondylolisthesis.

Q: How would you make this decision?

Traditionally this problem has been treated with decompressive laminectomy and fusion. In 1991 a landmark randomized controlled trial (RCT) by Herkowitz et al. demonstrated that patients undergoing decompressive laminectomy and fusion had significant improvements in clinical outcome. Following another RCT in 1997 by Fischgrund et al. showing similar outcomes, decompression and instrumented fusion became the treatment of choice and remained so for many years. However, several large studies with conflicting results subsequently caused further controversy. Now these cases are viewed more from the point of view of stability. Features that would encourage me to include a fusion in the surgery include sagittal facet orientation (loss of buttressing effect), facet effusions, absence of stabilising signs, younger patient and significant slippage upon weight-bearing.

SUGGESTED READINGS

1. Herkowitz HN, Kurtz LT. Degenerative lumbar spondylolisthesis with spinal stenosis: a prospective study comparing decompression with decompression and intertransverse process arthrodesis. J Bone Joint Surg Am. 1991;73(6):802–8.
2. Fischgrund JS, Mackay M, Herkowitz HN, et al. 1997 Volvo Award winner in clinical studies. Degenerative lumbar spondylolisthesis with spinal stenosis: a prospective, randomized study comparing decompressive laminectomy and arthrodesis with and without spinal instrumentation. Spine. 1997;22(24):2807–12.
3. Simmonds AM, Rampersaud YR, Dvorak MF, et al. Defining the inherent stability of degenerative spondylolisthesis: a systematic review. J Neurosurg Spine. 2015;23:178–89.

24

OPLL

You are asked to see a 64-year-old male who had emigrated from Japan 10 years previously. He presents with a long-standing history of neck pain but reports progressively worsening grip strength, manual dexterity, and unsteadiness when walking, over the past 4 months.

He is a type 2 diabetic and a non-smoker. On examination of his upper limbs, he has normal tone, with bilateral Medical Research Council (MRC) grade 4 power. He has objective weakness on grip strength assessment bilaterally, as well as difficulty picking up small objects such as a key and a coin.

He is hyper-reflexic on deep tendon reflex testing of the upper limb (biceps [C5/6], brachioradialis [C6] and triceps [C7]). He has patchy sensory deficits in both arms, without a defined dermatomal distribution and complains of intermittent tingling in his fingertips. Hoffman's sign and Romberg test are positive, with wide-based ataxia noted on gait assessment.

Q: How would you investigate this patient?

This patient demonstrates clinical signs of cervical myelopathy. I would request X-rays of the cervical spine (AP and lateral) to evaluate the sagittal alignment of the cervical spine. I would also request an MRI scan. A CT scan of the cervical spine would allow me to exclude ossification of either the PLL or the OLF. If these were normal, I would also perform an upper limb nerve conduction study to exclude peripheral neuropathy as a cause of the symptoms.

Q: What is the diagnosis?

The images confirm a diagnosis of cervical stenosis because of ossification of the posterior longitudinal ligament.

The lateral X-ray (Figure 24.1) shows multilevel ossification in the region of the PLL (see arrows), as well as anterior osteophytes/ossification of the anterior longitudinal ligament (ALL). The sagittal CT scan of the cervical spinal (Figure 24.2) shows diffuse ossification

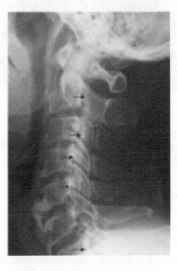

Figure 24.1 X-ray (lateral) cervical spine showing signs of ossification of posterior longitudinal ligament (marked).

DOI: 10.1201/9781003201304-26

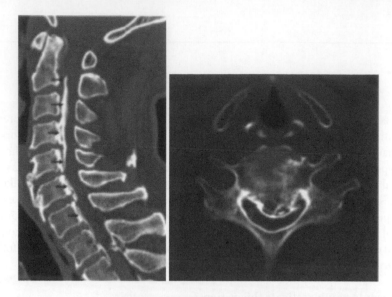

Figure 24.2a and b   CT scan cervical spine sagittal and axial (C4/5) showing OPLL of entire cervical spine.

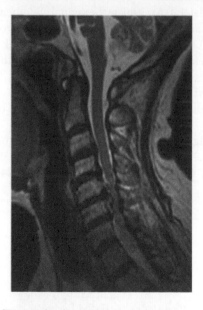

Figure 24.3   Sagittal MRI scan (T2-weighted) cervical spine showing cervical stenosis, maximal at C4–7.

from C2 to C7, causing stenosis of the cervical canal. The T2-weighted sagittal MRI image (Figure 24.3) shows resultant cord compression from C3–6.

Q: What is the pathophysiology of this condition?

OPLL is mostly found in men, the elderly and Far East Asian patients. The most affected levels are between C4 and C6 and 95% of the ossification is in the C spine.

There are several diseases associated with OPLL, such as DISH, AS, and other spondyloarthropathies. Genetic, hormonal, environmental and lifestyle factors have been reported to be associated with OPLL formation and progression. These include diabetes, obesity, a high salt–low meat diet and poor calcium absorption. However, the pathogenesis of OPLL is still unclear. Most symptomatic patients with OPLL present with neurological deficits such as myelopathy, radiculopathy and/or bowel and bladder symptoms.

Q: How would you manage this patient?

Non-operative management is reserved for non-symptomatic patients, with OPLL often diagnosed incidentally.

Most patients require surgical management with decompression ± fixation. This can be achieved through an anterior or posterior approach, depending on the extent of the spinal cord compression and shape of the cervical spine. **Anterior corpectomy with or without OPLL resection is** indicated in patients with kyphotic cervical spine.

Posterior laminectomy (removal of the whole lamina) or laminoplasty (removal of a section of the lamina) surgeries occasionally fail to relieve anterior compression of the spinal cord caused by preoperatively existing cervical kyphosis and/or OPLL. These anterior components prevent neurological recovery because the posterior decompression mechanism depends on the posterior drift back of the spinal cord.

Compared with the anterior approach, the posterior approach is less technically demanding and more applicable to multi-segmental lesions, which are often the case in OPLL patients. A decision regarding anterior versus posterior surgery can be helped by the use of the modified K line (Figure 24.4).

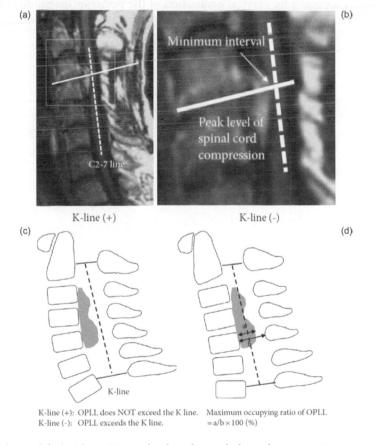

Figure 24.4a–d Modified K-line. T1-weighted midsagittal slice of preoperative magnetic resonance imaging showing the placement of the (a) K (C2–7) line (b) enlarged image. The arrow indicates the minimum interval at the peak level of spinal cord compression (c) K-line (+) and (d) K-line (−).

K+ patients can be managed via a posterior approach, while K− patients should be managed via anterior approaches.

Given the severity of this patient's symptoms, I would manage this patient surgically, via a posterior laminectomy and fusion with lateral mass screws.

Several factors have been reported to be associated with good surgical outcomes, including lordotic alignment of the cervical spine, preoperative morbidity less than 1 year, less compression of the spinal cord, OPLL with a diameter of less than 60% of the spinal canal, no history of trauma, lesser age, and less postoperative range of motion of the cervical spine.

SUGGESTED READINGS

1. Matsumoto M, Chiba K, Toyama Y. Surgical treatment of ossification of the posterior longitudinal ligament and its outcomes: posterior surgery by laminoplasty. Spine (Phila Pa 1976). 2012;37(5):E303–8.
2. Wu JC, Chen YC, Huang WC. Ossification of the posterior longitudinal ligament in cervical spine: prevalence, management, and prognosis. Neurospine. 2018;15(1):33–41.
3. Fujiyoshi T, Yamazaki M, Kawabe J, et al. A new concept for making decisions regarding the surgical approach for cervical ossification of the posterior longitudinal ligament: the K-line. Spine (Phila Pa 1976). 2008;33(26):E990–3.

SECTION 3
SPINAL CORD INJURY

25

INCOMPLETE SPINAL CORD INJURY

Q: A 31-year-old patient is admitted to the ER with progressive symptoms of right-sided lower extremity weakness and altered gait over the last 2 months. He also complains of thoracic pain. He is otherwise fit and well, on no regular medications, and works as a teacher. How do you proceed?

The weakness and altered gait may be due to neural compression either peripheral or central. The differential at this stage however is broad including tumour, infection and demyelinating disorders. I would therefore like to take a full history and examine the patient, focusing specifically on any signs of myelopathy. I would like to arrange appropriate imaging, depending on the full history and examination findings.

Q: Examination reveals the patient has Medical Research Council (MRC) grade 3/5 power, proprioceptive and fine-touch loss in his right lower limb. Motor power in the left lower limb is normal, but pinprick testing reveals loss of sensation throughout all dermatomes. A CT thoracic spine is arranged which is shown in the following image. Can you comment on the likely diagnosis?

The examination findings are consistent with a Brown–Sequard syndrome. The CT shows a parasagittal image showing multiple calcified thoracic discs—one of more of which are

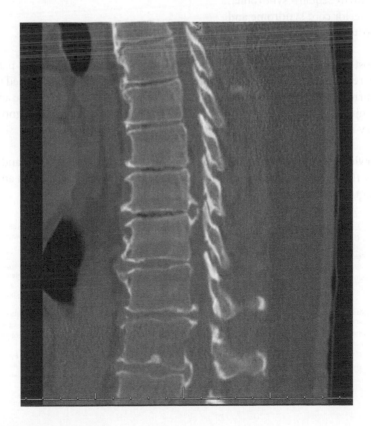

DOI: 10.1201/9781003201304-28

likely to have caused unilateral cord compression and this resulting pattern of injury. The pattern of deficit is due to dorsal column compression causing ipsilateral loss of fine touch, vibration, two-point discrimination and conscious proprioception. Disruption of the spinothalamic tracts causing contralateral pain, the temperature is due to the crossing of the tracts to the contralateral side after initially ascending a level. The ipsilateral weakness is caused by compression of the corticospinal tracts. At the level of the lesion, the pattern of weakness would be lower motor neurone weakness, and distal to this would be upper motor neurone weakness. Other causes of Brown–Sequard syndrome include penetrating trauma (e.g. stabbing), tumour and blunt trauma.

Q: MRI scan imaging of the neural axis confirms no other causes for the symptoms. How would you proceed?

Scrutiny of the imaging would be required to identify the compressive level. Surgical decompression would be required to prevent further worsening of symptoms but is associated with significant risks and would need careful counselling with the patient. Supportive multidisciplinary care and rehabilitation in the context of cord injury would also be required. Nonetheless, the prognosis is very good in terms of functional outcome.

Exam Tips

1. Incomplete spinal cord injuries are injuries with some preservation of function below the level of the injury. The classic injury patterns are

   - central cord syndrome (see q. 26),
   - Brown–Sequard syndrome,
   - anterior cord syndrome and
   - posterior cord syndrome (very rare).

The most common is central cord syndrome, most commonly in elderly patients caused by hyperextension mechanisms. Anterior cord syndrome is typically caused by hyperflexion injuries resulting in compression of the anterior cord and may involve anterior spinal artery injury, which supplies the anterior 2/3 of the spinal cord. The prognosis for motor recovery is very poor.

2. Knowledge of the arrangement of the ascending and descending tracts and the ability to draw them in cross section is highly recommended in the FRCS exam and a common viva question.

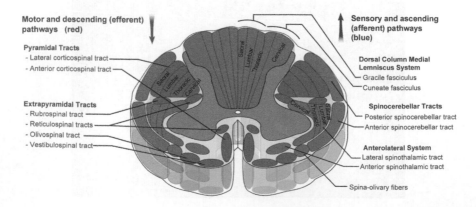

26

CENTRAL CORD SYNDROME

Q: A 57-year-old-male is admitted at midnight having fallen from a height of 6 feet whilst walking, landing heavily on his face. He suffered no loss of consciousness but experienced transient quadriparesis at the scene which has slowly improved. He complains of mild neck pain. CT scan imaging is as follows:

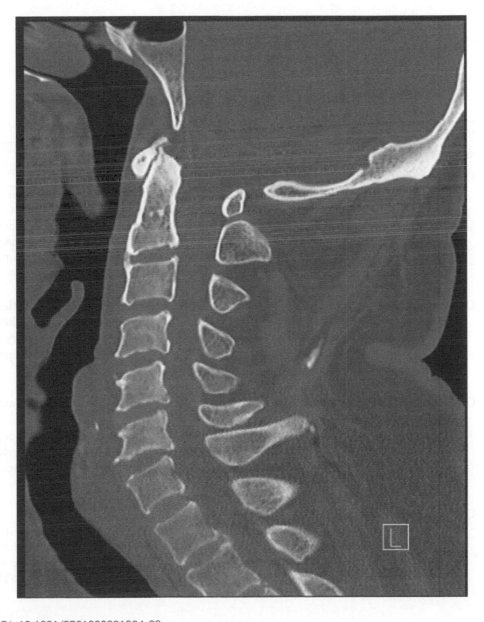

DOI: 10.1201/9781003201304-29

Motor Exam:

	Right	Left
C5	3	3
C6	1	2
C7	2	2
C8	0	0
T1	0	0

	Right	Left
L2	3	3
L3	4	4
L4	4	4
L5	3	2
S1	3	3

Q: What pattern of injury does this represent?

The most significant deficit is clearly in the upper limbs with almost normally preserved power in the lower limbs. The upper extremity motor scores are more than 10 Medical Research Council (MRC) points lower than the lower extremity motor scores and therefore qualifies as a central cord injury. The hyperextension injury suggested in the history is typical in the elderly population. Hyperextension causes buckling of the ligamentum flavum, cord compression and axonal injury.

Q: Why are the upper extremities affected more profoundly than the lower extremities?

This was originally thought to be due to the anatomical somatotrophy. This is now, however, thought not to be the case and considered to be due to corticospinal tracts subserving more fine movements, especially in hand function, so functional deficits in distal upper extremities are more pronounced.

Q: The patient has an American Spinal Cord Injury Association (ASIA) C injury. How would you proceed?

There would appear to be no obvious identifiable fracture on this patient's CT, although this is only a single CT slice, but the patient has likely suffered an injury to the cervical cord. I would like to organise an urgent MRI scan to assess his cord as well as the presence of any discoligamentous injury.

Q: The MRI is as shown. Can you comment?

This is a sagittal T2-weighted image of this patient's cervical spine. It is suggestive of increased T2 cord signal from C3–C7. Multilevel degenerative disc disease and flaval infolding have resulted in multilevel stenosis. There does not appear to be any disco-ligamentous injury on the MRI, although I would like to examine the STIR sequence.

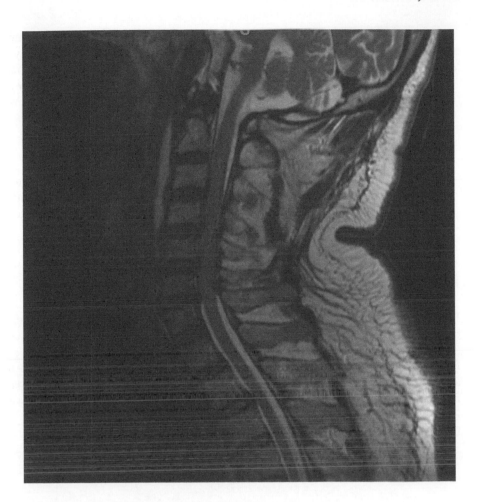

Q: How would you treat this patient?

The treatment of central cord injuries remains controversial. As a general rule I would treat American Spinal Cord Injury Association (ASIA) C injuries operatively and American Spinal Cord Injury Association (ASIA) D injuries, particularly if improving neurologically, non-operatively. Three factors that I would consider when making this decision are (1) ongoing cord compression, (2) neurology and (3) stability. If there is ongoing cord compression, the patient requires urgent decompression. If the patient is continuing to improve neurologically, then observation may be reasonable. If there is any question of instability, the patient requires stabilisation. In this patient, although there is some suggestion that neurologically they are improving, there is clear ongoing compression evident on the scan, and I would therefore like to treat this patient surgically.

Q: What operation would you like to perform?

The patient has multilevel spinal stenosis with ongoing compression. I would perform either a decompressive laminectomy and fusion or a laminoplasty procedure.

Q: When would you take this patient to theatre, and why?

In 2012 a prospective cohort study performed across 6 North American centres with 313 patients (STASCIS study) compared early versus delayed decompression in acute spinal cord injury (SCI) showed that the odds of at least a 2 grade improvement in American

Spinal Cord Injury Association (ASIA) Impairment Scale were 2.8 times higher amongst those who underwent early (<24h) compared to late (>24h) decompression. They concluded decompression after SCI prior to 24h can be performed safely and is associated with improved neurological outcome. The 2017 AO guidelines suggest early surgery (24h) should be considered in traumatic central cord syndrome (TCCS). On this basis, I would take the patient to theatre within 24h.

Exam Tip

- Central cord syndrome is a common presentation following trauma, particularly in the elderly. A structured approach to assessment of the neurological findings and consideration of the reasons to operate as listed earlier will form the basis for an excellent answer.

SUGGESTED READINGS

1. Fehlings M, Vaccaro A, Wilson JR, et al. Early versus delayed decompression for traumatic cervical spinal cord injury: results of the surgical timing in acute spinal cord injury study (STASCIS). PLoS ONE. 2012;7(2):e32037.
2. Fehlings M, Tetreault LA, Wilson JR, et al. A clinical practice guideline for the management of patients with acute spinal cord injury and central cord syndrome: recommendations on the timing (<24h v >24h) of decompressive surgery. Global Spine J. 2017;7(3 Suppl):195S–202S.

27

COMPLETE SPINAL CORD INJURY

Q: A 28-year-old-male, motorcycle RTA at 80kph. He was reported as unable to move or feel his legs at the scene but moving both arms voluntarily. GCS 14. Haemodynamically stable throughout. His thoracic spine trauma CT is shown below. Can you comment?

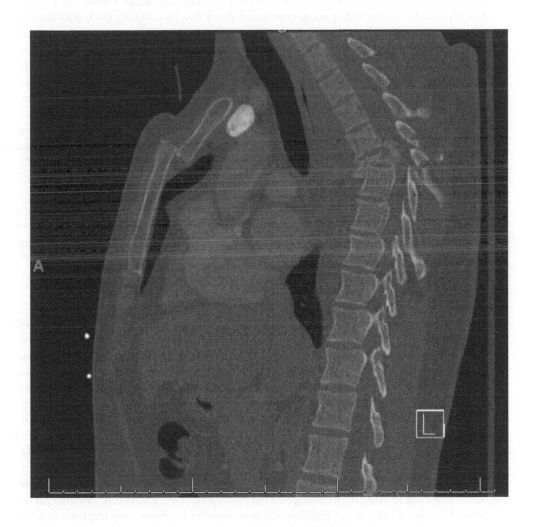

The CT scan shows a severely comminuted burst fracture of the upper thoracic spine, likely around the T5 level. The fracture appears to extend posteriorly, and there is significant kyphosis at this level. There is retropulsion of the fracture fragments which would be concerning for a severe thoracic cord injury. I also note that there is a displaced sternal fracture which adds to the instability of this already highly unstable fracture.

Q: The CT shows that his other injuries include multiple rib fractures (no flail), left apical pneumothorax and right frontal lobe contusion. He has been assessed by the trauma team, and a chest drain has been inserted. There is no neurosurgical concern regarding his contusion. How do you proceed?

This patient has suffered a major trauma, which is concern for a complete cord injury. I would first assess him clinically. He is currently haemodynamically stable, but I would nonetheless determine if the patient is in spinal shock first by checking the bulbocavernosus reflex. I would perform a full assessment according to the American Spinal Cord Injury Association (ASIA) grading system. This involves an assessment of bilateral motor function in upper and lower limbs, followed by a sensory assessment to both pinprick and light touch again in both upper and lower limbs. This would then be followed by logroll and sensory testing to the sacral dermatomes, and deep anal pressure (DAP) and voluntary anal contraction (VAC) assessment. I would then follow the American Spinal Cord Injury Association (ASIA) guidelines for determining the sensory and motor levels, the neurological level of injury and whether the injury is complete or incomplete. I would then establish the overall American Spinal Cord Injury Association (ASIA) impairment scale.

Q: Your assessment shows that this is a complete injury. What does this mean?

A complete spinal cord injury (SCI) means that there is no sacral sparing. This is defined by the absence of VAC, absence of any sensation in the S4–S5 dermatomes and absent DAP. The implications of this are that the prognosis is very poor in terms of functional recovery.

Q: How would you proceed with the management of this patient and in what time period?

This is a highly unstable injury and requires surgical stabilisation, decompression and restoration of spinal alignment. The 2012 STASCIS study by Fehlings et al. demonstrated that decompression prior to 24h after SCI is associated with improved neurological outcome. I would therefore like to take the patient to the theatre as an urgent case on the next available emergency list. I would obtain an MRI scan to assess for epidural haematoma and the site of greatest compression. The patient requires an anaesthetic assessment due to the concern regarding his chest injury and pneumothorax, especially given that he would be lying prone. The cardiothoracic team would need to be consulted given his sternal injury as, given the displacement, it may require fixation and cardiac monitoring.

Once intubated, the patient may benefit from a 'sandwich flip' technique on the Jackson table rather than a standard logroll, given the instability of the fracture, in order to get the patient safely into the prone position. Once prone, the kyphosis may improve to some degree but would need to be checked with inter-operative imaging, either XR or CT. The patient then requires a two up–two down construct with thoracic pedicle screws and rods in order to stabilise the spine. I would then perform a laminectomy at the injury level in order to decompress the cord and facilitate the best chance of recovery.

Q: Is this patient likely to recover any motor function?

The prognosis for this patient unfortunately remains very poor in terms of recovery of function. Approximately 80% of patients may improve one nerve root level and 20%, two root levels. Current research suggests time-specific biomarkers can describe acute SCI which have potential in injury stratification and possibly predicting outcome.

Exam Tips

- In any potential cord injury case in the FRCS, always assess according to Advanced Trauma and Life Support (ATLS) principles maintaining spinal precautions to protect the cord. Always bear in mind the associated injuries that may exist and be a potentially greater risk to the patient in the short term than, for example, pneumothorax in this case.
- Assessment using the American Spinal Cord Injury Association (ASIA) system is the next key step, and determination of whether the injury is complete or not. The STASCIS study demonstrated decompression prior to 24h after SCI is associated with improved neurological outcome. Further studies using the STASCIS data have since shown severe American Spinal Cord Injury Association (ASIA) grade at initial presentation to be associated with a greater likelihood of complications and that early decompression is more cost-effective.

SUGGESTED READINGS

1. Fehlings M, Vaccaro A, Wilson JR, et al. Early versus delayed decompression for traumatic cervical spinal cord injury: results of the surgical timing in acute spinal cord injury study (STASCIS). PLoS ONE. 2012;7(2):e32037.
2. Badhiwala J, Ahuja C, Fehlings M. Time is spine: a review of translational advances in spinal cord injury. J Neurosurg Spine. 2018;30(1):1–18.
3. Kwon BK, Bloom O, Wanner I-B, et al. Neurochemical biomarkers in spinal cord injury. Spinal Cord. 2019;57(10):819–31.

SECTION 4
SPINAL DEFORMITY

28

ADULT DEGENERATIVE SCOLIOSIS

Q: The X-ray (XR) below shows a 71-year-old patient who comes to see you in clinic with a chief complaint of lumbar mechanical back pain and right leg pain. Can you comment on the XRs?

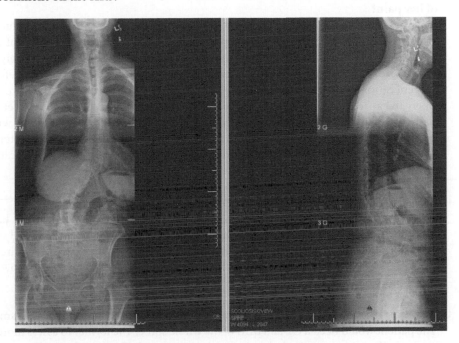

This is an AP and lateral 36-inch standing XR. The coronal view demonstrates a right-sided lumbar scoliosis with an apex at the L3/4 disc. There is marked loss of coronal alignment. The sagittal view demonstrates the patient stands in positive sagittal balance. There appears to be loss of lumbar lordosis and a spondylolisthesis at L5/S1.

Q: Are you aware of any specific measurements that may be helpful when attempting to assess this patient?

On the AP XR, I would assess the coronal balance by marking the C7 plumb line and the central sacral vertical line. On the lateral XR, I would assess sagittal balance using the C7 plumb line assessing how far anterior it passes to the posterosuperior aspect of S1. I would like to measure the magnitude of the curves using the Cobb angle. I would also like to measure the total lumbar lordosis between the upper endplate of L1 and S1 which in the normal patient should approximately 40 degrees. I would also measure the pelvic incidence, pelvic tilt and sacral slope. The pelvic incidence is the angle between a line perpendicular to the sacral endplate at its midpoint and a line connecting this point to the femoral head axis. This should approximate to the lumbar lordosis +/−10 degrees. Furthermore, the following equation should be satisfied:

$$PI = SS + PT$$

DOI: 10.1201/9781003201304-32

These measurements will help to identify the key issues that need addressing in any formal corrective procedure. These measurements will also then help classify the deformity according to the SRS–Scwabb classification system.

Q: The patient had good relief from repeated right L5 nerve root blocks over the past 3 years. Examination reveals she has Gr 3/5 weakness in her right extensor hallucis longus, otherwise neurologically intact. Past medical history is positive for hypertension and gastroesophageal reflux disease. She is looking for a more definitive solution for both her leg pain and back pain. Can you suggest the aetiology of her pain?

This patient has adult degenerative scoliosis. Her right leg pain is likely due to L5 nerve root entrapment secondary to spinal or foraminal stenosis as a result of degenerative changes or vertebral rotation or translation. Her back pain is likely to be multifactorial resulting from the degenerative cascade that has led to her deformity. Degeneration of the discs and segmental instability, such as at L5/S1 in this case, are likely to cause pain. Facetal pain may contribute, arising from degenerate facets. Back pain can also arise from postural imbalance, often referred to as being out with the 'cone of economy' as described by Dubousset. Muscular effort is much greater when this cone is exceeded. There may be additional stress placed on the sacroiliac and hip joints, causing further pain.

Q: What may be the definitive solution to her problems?

This patient requires adult scoliosis correction to address multiple issues. The key surgical goals would be to re-establish spinopelvic alignment, correct sagittal and coronal deformity, decompress the neural elements and achieve fusion. This would require a long construct with interbody fusions and spinal osteotomies, most likely from the lower thoracic spine to the pelvis.

Q: What further investigations might you carry out in your pre-operative assessment?

The patient would need a CT and MRI of the whole spine. The former to assess more accurately the bony anatomy and plan screw placement and, if required, spinal osteotomies. The latter would help to assess nerve root compression and position of the cord/cauda equina through the region of the correction. Bending films will help assessment of the flexibility of the spine and help to plan the proximal extent of the construct.

Exam Tips

- The exam focus on an adult spinal deformity case is in the global assessment of the spinal deformity rather than specifics of the corrective procedure required: knowledge of how to assess sagittal and coronal balance and spino-pelvic parameters and interpret them will form an excellent basis for your answer. Defining the key surgical goals in a case such as the preceding one is far better than describing a specific operation.
- If presented with a case of adult spinal deformity, consider that the aetiology will be one of three main types (as described by Aebi et al.): **primary degenerative** scoliosis that develops after skeletal maturity, predominantly affects lumbar spine and results from the degenerative cascade described earlier; **idiopathic** scoliosis that develops before skeletal maturity but becomes symptomatic in adult life (not confined to lumbar spine); or **secondary degenerative** scoliosis which is scoliosis secondary to other pathology such as hip pathology or metabolic bone disease.

REFERENCE

Vialle LR, Lenke LG, Cheung KMC. AOSpine masters series; Volume 4: adult spinal deformities. New York, NY: Thieme; 2015.

29

SCHEUERMANN'S KYPHOSIS

You are asked to see a 22-year-old male with a long-standing history of back pain related to what he describes as a humpback (Figure 29.1). This was first diagnosed in adolescence but had been gradually progressive over the past 2–3 years.

He complains of worsening breathing difficulties which he feels are related to his spinal deformity, and he complains of psychological concerns related to the shape of his back.

A plain radiograph (Figure 29.2) and CT scan (Figure 29.3) of the whole spine were performed.

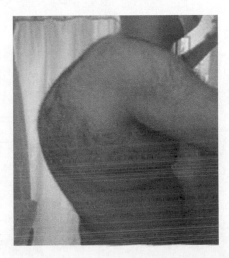

Figure 29.1 Clinical photograph showing patient with Scheuermann's kyphosis.

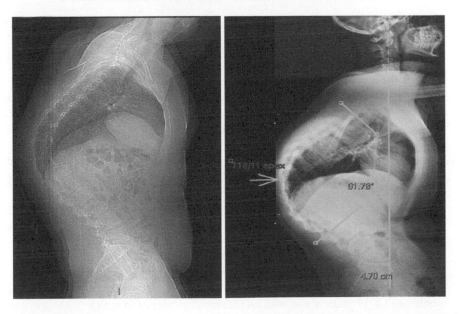

Figure 29.2 Lateral whole-spine X-ray showing thoracic kyphosis of 92 degrees with an apex at T10/11.

DOI: 10.1201/9781003201304-33

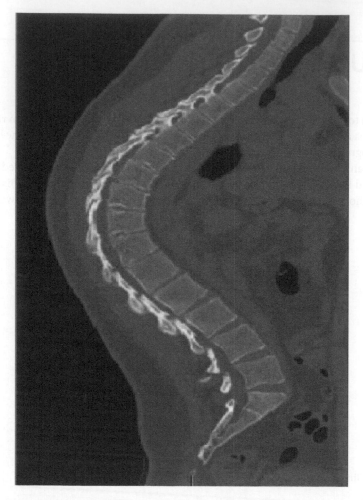

Figure 29.3   CT scan (sagittal view) whole spine showing thoracic kyphosis with an apex at T10/11.

Q: What is the most likely diagnosis?

The history and imaging are suggestive of Scheuermann's kyphosis. This is a rigid thoracic hyper-kyphosis defined by a greater than 45-degree curve caused by >5 degree anterior wedging across three consecutive vertebrae with narrowing of the intervertebral disc spaces.

It is the most common structural kyphosis in adolescents. Whilst its exact aetiology is unknown, genetic, hormonal and mechanical influences have been implicated, including

- osteonecrosis of the anterior apophyseal ring,
- altered biomechanics leading to anterior biomechanics leading to anterior wedging and subsequent growth arrest and
- relative osteoporosis leading to anterior compression deformity.

Autosomal dominant inheritance pattern has now been accepted. Typical age of onset is between 10–13 years of age, with an increased incidence in males.

Mild curves (<70 degrees) cause back pain that rarely limits daily activities. Curves above 75 degrees are likely to cause thoracic pain, while more severe curves above 100 degrees can be associated with pulmonary issues.

Q: What are the classical features of Scheuermann's kyphosis on plain X-ray?

- On X-ray whole spine (lateral)
  - Anterior wedging across three consecutive vertebrae >5 degrees
  - Disc space narrowing
  - Endplate irregularities including Schmorl's nodes (disc herniation into vertebral endplate)
  - Compensatory lumbar hyper-lordosis
  - Spondylolysis on dedicated lumbar films if the patient has low back pain
- On X-ray whole spine (AP)
  - Scoliosis
- Supine lateral radiograph with the patient lying in hyperextension over a bolster can help differentiate from postural from structural kyphosis
  - Scheuermann's kyphosis usually relatively inflexible on bending radiograph

Q: How can this condition be classified?

- Thoracic Scheuermann's kyphosis
  - Most common form
  - Curve from T1/2 to T12/L1 with apex between T6–T8
  - Better prognosis
- Thoracolumbar/lumbar Scheuermann's kyphosis
  - Less common form
  - Curve from T4/5 to L2/3 with apex near the thoracolumbar junction
  - Associated with increased back pain
  - More likely to be progressive.

This patient is affected by thoracolumbar Scheuermann's kyphosis.

Q: Is further imaging required?

CT scanning is not routinely required but can be useful for surgical planning (Figure 29.3). The use of MRI in patients without neurological symptoms is controversial. It can be useful to identify associated disc herniation, epidural cysts, spinal cord abnormalities and spinal stenosis. The presence of neurological symptoms is an absolute indication for diagnostic MRI.

Q: How should this condition be treated?

The treatment algorithm for SK can be broken up into 3 key decisions:

a Determination of whether the patient's clinical picture warrants intervention
b Determination of whether they require operative or non-operative management
c Selection of treatment approach

Non-operative management (observation and physiotherapy) is indicated in most patients with less severe curves (<60 degrees) and mild symptoms.

Extension braces can be effective in moderate kyphosis (60–80 degrees) in patients with growth potential remaining. Research has shown poor adherence with bracing in adolescence due to concerns regarding cosmesis.

Indications for operative management include

- severity of deformity (>80 degrees),
- neurological deficit,
- spinal cord compression and
- patient age—older patients are likely to have less flexible, more severe (>80 degree) curves.

Modern surgical techniques are primarily posterior (Figure 29.4), with additional anterior release being associated with significant morbidity and necessary only in the most severe curves. Pedicle subtraction osteotomy (PSO) and Smith Peterson Osteotomy (SPO) can be used to improve the degree of surgical correction (See spinal osteotomy q. 30.)

Q: What are the risks of deformity correction surgery?
These include

- neurological complications (typically due to spinal cord stretching/lengthening,
- distal and proximal junctional kyphosis (14–26%) and
- pseudoarthrosis, hardware failure (22–25%), loss of correction and so on.

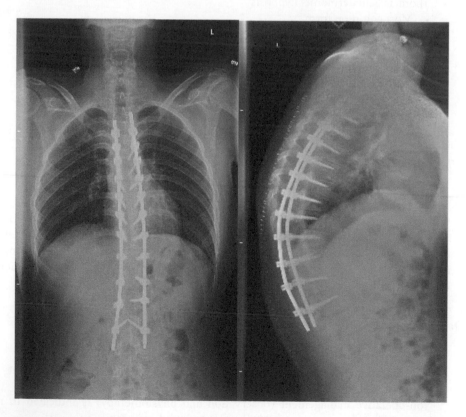

Figure 29.4   Plain radiographs (AP and lateral whole spine) after posterior instrumented correction and fusion of thoracic kyphosis.

Intraoperative neuromonitoring (IONM; See spinal cord monitoring q. 49) has become increasingly prevalent in spinal deformity surgery over the past several decades, and multimodal monitoring should be implemented during surgical correction.

Exam Tip

- You should be aware of the basic parameters used to assess balance in the spine, as well as how to draw the CSVL (central sacral vertical line) and PSVL (posterior sacral vertical line; Figure 29.5) The PSVL allows for the identification of the sagittal stable vertebra, which is needed to identify the best levels for instrumentation. The paper by Sardar et al. (included in the references) is an excellent and comprehensive summary on this topic.

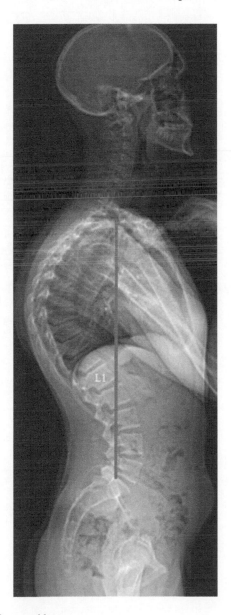

Figure 29.5 Posterior sacral vertical line.

SUGGESTED READINGS

1.   Haq S, Ehresman J, Cottrill E, et al. Treatment approaches for Scheuermann kyphosis: a systematic review of historic and current management. J Neurosurg Spine. 2019;32(2):235–47.
2.   Ali RM, Green DW, Patel TC. Scheuermann's kyphosis. Curr Opin Pediatr. 1999;11:70–5.
3.   Sardar Z, Ames RJ, Lenke L. Scheuermann's kyphosis: diagnosis, management, and selecting fusion levels. J Am Acad Orthop Surg. 2019;27(10):e462–72.

30

SPINAL OSTEOTOMY

Q: A 42-year-old-male attends your clinic complaining of worsening thoracic pain. His sagittal X-ray (XR) follows. Can you comment on the XR?

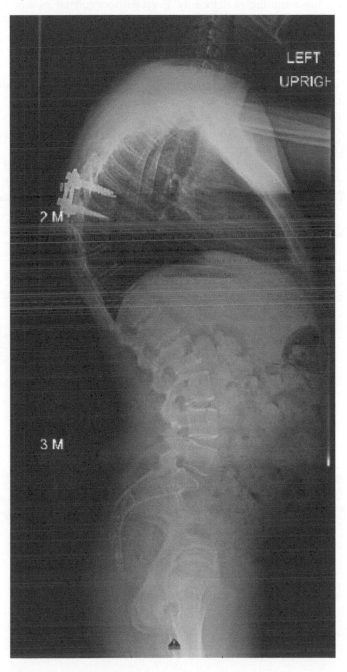

This is a 36-inch standing sagittal view which demonstrates a significant kyphosis, centred at approximately T9. There is evidence of a short segment screw and rod construct. I would like to formally measure thoracic kyphosis. Normal kyphosis is between 25 and 40 degrees. His most likely diagnosis is Scheuermann's kyphosis.

Q: This patient does indeed have Scheuermann's kyphosis. He has had multiple fusion procedures which have failed to adequately correct his deformity. Can you suggest what may be required next to address this?

This patient has a significant deformity. Even without formal measurement, this looks to be of the order of 90 degrees. The T9 level itself has a significant kyphosis. Given the magnitude of the kyphosis, he would most likely need one or multiple spinal osteotomies in order to correct this.

Q: Can you describe a spinal osteotomy and are you aware of any associated classification systems?

In 2014, Schwab et al. described the comprehensive anatomical spinal osteotomy classification system of spinal osteotomies to address rigid deformity patterns. This system describes 6 osteotomy subtypes graded from 1–6.

Grade 1 is a partial facet joint resection; grade 2 is a complete facet joint resection (equivalent to a Smith–Petersen osteotomy) with the correction through the disc space. Grade 3 is a pedicle and partial body resection (equivalent to a pedicle subtraction osteotomy). Grade 5 involves complete resection of the vertebra and discs (vertebral column resection).

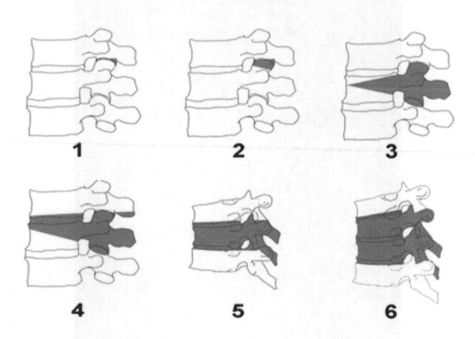

Q: How much correction can be achieved with these osteotomies?

A Smith–Pietersen osteotomy can achieve up to 10 degrees. A PSO can achieve 30–40 degrees of correction. VCR, including multiple levels, can achieve larger corrections still. Great care must be taken when performing these procedures to avoid excessive kinking/traction of the cord and causing a subsequent cord injury, and I would use interoperative spinal cord monitoring to mitigate the risk of this.

Exam Tip

- A detailed knowledge of spinal osteotomies is not required for the FRCS exam, but an awareness of the grading system and that they can be used to achieve progressively larger deformity corrections is useful information to add to any question on spinal deformity. An awareness of the risk to the cord at the moment of correction is paramount and is increased with larger osteotomies.

SUGGESTED READINGS

1. Schwab F, Blondel B, Chay E, et al. The comprehensive anatomical spinal osteotomy classification. Neurosurgery. 2014;74(1):112–20.
2. Kose KC, Bozduman O, Yenigul AE, et al. Spinal osteotomies: indications, limits and pitfalls. EFORT Open Rev. 2017;2(3):73–82.

31

ADULT ISTHMIC SPONDYLOLISTHESIS

You are referred a 46-year-old male from his GP. He has a history of back pain which started in his late teens and was exacerbated after a fall from standing height 6 months ago.

Since the fall, he complains of worsening bilateral lateral calf pain which he describes as being 'burning' in nature. He is a keen gym-goer, but his pain has stopped him being able to exercise. He denies any abnormal bowel or bladder symptoms.

On examination, he has an antalgic gait. He has Medical Research Council (MRC) grade 5 power throughout his upper and lower limbs, except for slight right-sided weakness in ankle and great toe dorsiflexion. Muscle tone is normal. He has bilaterally reduced sensation to light touch over his lateral calf. He has normal reflex testing and plantar reflexes are down-going.

Q: What investigations would you order for this patient?

I would obtain AP and lateral views of the lumbar spine (Figure 31.1), as well as an MRI scan of the lumbar spine (Figure 31.2). Standing lateral flexion-extension radiographs of the lumbar spine help diagnose dynamic instability (spondylolisthesis) and can identify defects (fractures) in the pars interarticularis. In the absence of a reliable diagnosis on plain radiographs, a CT scan is considered the most reliable method of diagnosing a pars interarticularis defect (Figure 31.3).

MRI is the gold standard in the identification of canal stenosis or neural compression.

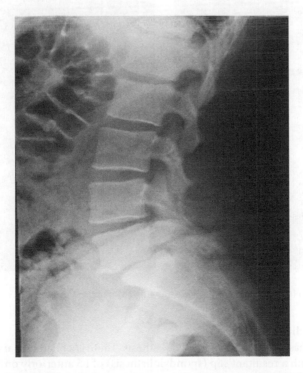

Figure 31.1   Plain radiograph (lateral) showing L5 pars defect and L5/S1 spondylolisthesis.

DOI: 10.1201/9781003201304-35

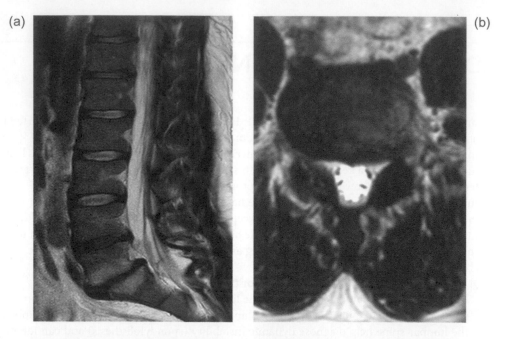

Figure 31.2 (a) T2-weighted MRI lumbar spine with (b) axial slice through L5/S1) showing bilateral foraminal stenosis, spondylolisthesis and severe endplate degeneration.

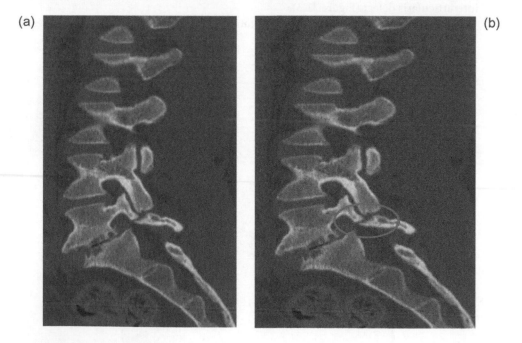

Figure 31.3 CT scan (a) lumbar spine marked showing (b) pars fracture.

Q: What is the diagnosis?

This patient has adult isthmic spondylolisthesis. There is a bilateral pars defect (spondylolysis) of L5 with a resultant slip (spondylolisthesis) of L5 anteriorly on S1. The MRI shows an associated compression of the exiting L5 neural foramina.

Q: How can this condition be classified?

The Wiltse classification divides spondylolisthesis into 5 groups (I–V):

- I Dysplastic: translation secondary to an abnormal neural arch
- II Isthmic (pars defect)
  - a—lytic (stress fracture; most common)
  - b—multiple injury/healing events leading to pars elongation
  - c—acute pars fracture (rare)
- III Degenerative
- IV Traumatic—acute posterior arch fracture (other than pars)
- V Neoplastic—pathological destruction of pars

The Meyering classification quantifies the amount of displacement of the slip of one vertebra on another:

- I <25%
- II 25–50%
- III 50–75%
- IV 75–100%
- V >100% (spondyloptysis)

Q: What is the cause of isthmic spondylolisthesis?

The cause of isthmic spondylolisthesis is thought to be multifactorial. The pars interarticularis is subject to maximal mechanical stress at the lumbosacral junction and the coronal orientation of the lower lumbar facet joints. In the lower lumbar spine, the cross-sectional anatomy of the pars is relatively thin.

A congenitally dysplastic pars combined with an increase in the forces concentrated across the pars with lumbar extension can lead to stress fractures. Repetitive stress from sports involving hyperextension, such as gymnastics and fast bowling (cricket), may result in the development of spondylolysis and spondylolisthesis. In the general adult population, the prevalence of asymptomatic adult isthmic spondylolisthesis has been estimated to be between 3.7–11.5%

Q: Can you outline the relevant lumbopelvic parameters on a lumbar spinal lateral plain radiograph? How are these linked to the incidence of this condition? (Figure 31.4)

Adult patients with isthmic spondylolisthesis generally have a higher pelvic incidence, sacral slope, pelvic tilt and lumbar lordosis. In isthmic spondylolisthesis, the defect in the pars interarticularis does not permit adequate load sharing in the posterior spinal elements (facet joints, lamina, etc.).

With the weight of the body vertically loading the spinal column because of the incompetence of the posterior elements, there is a shearing moment imparted to the intervertebral disc. The shear force can be amplified by local kyphosis and a dome-shaped sacrum. This can accelerate disc degeneration.

Q: How should this patient be managed?

Most patients can be managed non-operatively with analgesia (including neuropathic agents such as pregabalin and gabapentin), lifestyle modification and physiotherapy.

Surgical management is reserved for patients with persistent symptoms who have failed 6 months of non-operative management. Low-grade slips at L5/S1 (Meyerding I–II) can be managed either by posterior L5/S1 fusion (Figure 31.5) or ALIF. Both these procedures

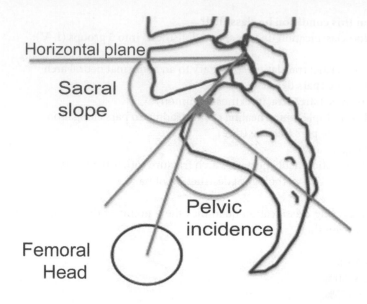

'X' delineates the mid-point of the sacral platform.

Figure 31.4   Key lumbopelvic parameters.

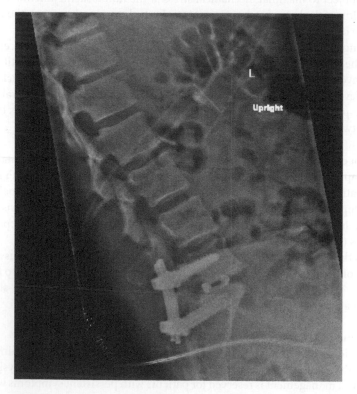

Figure 31.5   Lateral plain radiograph of the lumbar spine after posterior decompression and fusion with interbody cage (L5/S1).

aim to achieve interbody fusion. Posterior decompression and fusion procedures (PLIF/TLIF) directly decompress the neural elements, while anterior approaches such as the ALIF aim to achieve indirect foraminal decompression.

High-grade slips (Meyerding III and above) can often not be managed by ALIF due to the extreme angle of the L5/S1 disc space which makes anterior access difficult. Current evidence does not show better clinical outcomes following reduction and fixation of the slip versus fixation in situ.

Exam Tips

- Always think of a pars defect in younger patients with long-standing lower back pain.
- **Pelvic incidence (PI) = pelvic tilt (PT) + sacral slope (SS)**
- Normal PI is around 50 degrees normal PT is around 10–15 degrees, while normal SS is around 30–40 degrees.

SUGGESTED READINGS

1. Kalichman L, Kim, DH, Li L, et al. Spondylolysis and spondylolisthesis: prevalence and association with low back pain in the adult community-based population. Spine (Phila Pa 1976). 2009;34(2):199–205.

2. Lian X-F, Hou T-S, Xu J-G, et al. Single segment of posterior lumbar interbody fusion for adult isthmic spondylolisthesis: reduction or fusion in situ. Eur Spine J. 2014;23(1):172–9.

3. Bhalla A, Bono CM. Isthmic lumbar spondylolisthesis. Neurosurg Clin N Am. 2019;30(3):283–90.

32

DEFORMITY IN ANKYLOSING SPONDYLITIS

You are referred a 41-year-old male who presents to the spinal outpatient clinic with a significantly stooped posture. This had gradually increased in magnitude since his mid-20s.

He has a history of lumbosacral pain, which is most severe in the morning and reports a 2-year history of bilateral hip pain which is worsened by ambulation. His exercise tolerance is limited by exertional breathlessness after walking 200 yards on the flat.

On examination, he has a significant kyphotic deformity with a chin-on-chest deformity. He is neurologically intact with bilaterally normal upper and lower limb tone, power, reflexes, sensation and coordination.

Plain radiographs AP (Figure 32.1) and lateral of the pelvis, as well as cervical spine and standing views of the whole spine (AP and lateral; Figure 32.2), are requested.

Q: What is the most likely diagnosis?

The most likely diagnosis is AS. AS is a chronic inflammatory joint disease that predominantly affects the sacroiliac joints and spine. Differential diagnoses include DISH. AS is more likely given the age of the patient, the presence of bilateral sacroiliac joint fusion and bilateral hip osteoarthritis on pelvic radiograph.

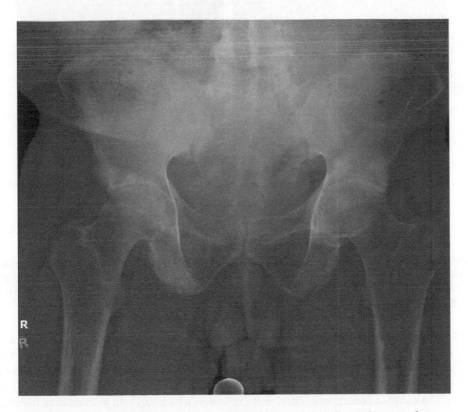

Figure 32.1 AP pelvic radiograph showing bilateral hip degeneration and sacroiliac joint fusion.

DOI: 10.1201/9781003201304-36

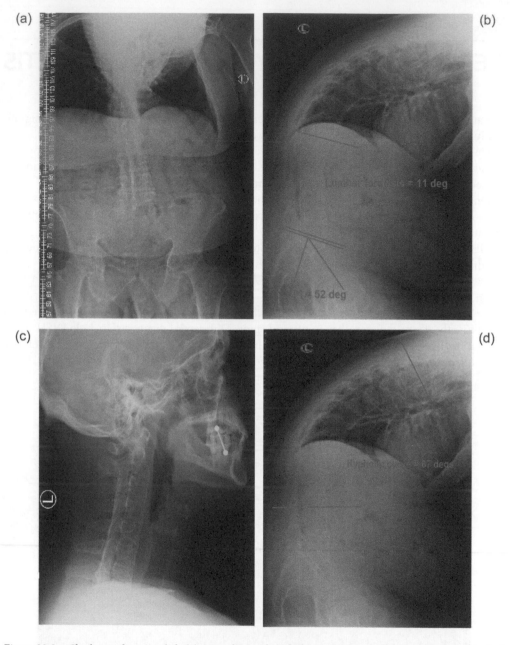

Figure 32.2 Clockwise from top left: (a) AP radiography whole spine (showing chin on chest deformity); (b) lateral thoracolumar spine radiograph showing 11-degree lumbar lordosis and 52 degrees of pelvic incidence; (c) lateral radiograph (whole spine) showing 67-degree kyphotic deformity; (d) later cervical spine plain radiograph showing joint ankylosis.

Other findings consistent with AS include symptoms onset in the 3rd decade of life, male gender (AS has a 4:1 M:F preponderence) and progressive spinal deformity (AS is associated with progressive thoracic kyphosis, which occurs due to multiple anteriorly wedged microfractures).

AS causes a reduction in chest wall expansion which can lead to exertional breathlessness. The classical spinal radiographic appearance in AS is described as a 'bamboo spine'

Table 32.1 Differences between DISH and AS

	Diffuse Idiopathic Skeletal Hyperostosis (DISH)	Ankylosing Spondylitis (AS)
Aetiology	Idiopathic	Autoimmune
Incidence	2.9-25%	0.05-1.4%
Age of onset	>45 years	<30
Sex ratio (M/F)	2:1	3:1
Clinical features	Pain, radiculopathy, dysphagia, risk of spinal and peripheral fractures	Pain, spinal stiffness, characteristic postural abnormalities (kyphosis), involvement of large peripheral joints
Radiological features	Affects anterior longitudinal ligament of the spine, spares intervertebral disc spaces and sacroiliac joints	Intervertebral and SI joint fusion
Laboratory investigations	Non specific and inconclusive	High ESR and CRP. Presence of HLA B27 (most cases)
Associated diseases	Obesity and diabetes mellitus	Autoimmune conditions like iritis, uveitis and ulcerative colitis
Treatment	Symptomatic	DMARDS, NSAIDS, surgery (rarely) for correction of spinal deformity of fracture fixation

appearance, with 'squaring' of vertebral bodies, osteopenia and ossifiction of intervertebral disc spaces.

Diagnostic criteria for AS are as follow:

- Bilateral sacroilitis
- ± uveitis
- HLA-B27 positivity

DISH is more commonly associated with older males, those with diabetes and radiographically spares in the intervertebral disc spaces. Sacroiliac joint involvement generally excludes a diagnosis of DISH, and patients may have increased radiodensity rather than the osteopenia seen in AS. (Table 32.1)

Q: How would you examine this patient?

I would perform a full upper and lower limb neurological examination, as well as a gait assessment to assess the functional impact of the patient's deformity. Specifically, sciatic nerve dysfunction should be identified. This can be due to piriformis spasm and can cause lower limb neuropathic symptoms.

The patient should be asked to stand upright against a flat surface. The cervico-thoracic or upper thoracic kyphosis deformity associated with severe AS can lead to a chin on chest deformity, with a loss of horizontal gaze. Costovertebral joint involvement can lead to reduced chest wall expansion, and patients should be inspected for signs of breathlessness after gait examination.

Pain on palpation of the cervicothoracic spine in AS should lead to a suspicion of fracture even if there has been no documented history of trauma. Schober's test is used to evaluate lumbar stiffness—with the patient standing, mark the skin overlying the 5th lumbar spinous process (usually at the level of the 'Dimples of Venus') and a level 10cm above. On forward flexion, this should increase to >15cm.

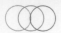

Sacroiliac joint involvement can be assessed by provocative tests which stress the joint, including the FABER test (flexion abduction external rotation of the ipsilateral hip causes pain) and direct palpation over the SI joint. Hip flexion contractures can be assessed by Thomas's test and with the patient in a supine and seated position. This helps differentiate sagittal plane imbalance due to hip flexion contractures rather than true kyphotic spinal deformity.

Q: What imaging and/or other investigations would you request?

Standing full-length AP and lateral of axial spine should be taken, but these have a poor sensitivity for occult fracture in AS. Classical findings include marginal syndesmophytes and late vertebral scalloping (bamboo spine; Figure 32.3).

CT scans are the most sensitive in detecting fracture in patients with AS, while MRI can be more useful in early AS, where enthesitis (inflammatory of soft tissue bony insertion) is predominant.

Blood tests have little diagnostic value in AS, while fluoroscopic or CT guided SI joint injections can be of diagnostic and therapeutic value.

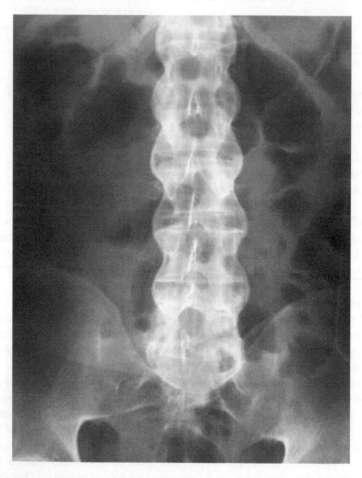

Figure 32.3 AP plain radiograph lumbar spine showing the characteristic 'Bamboo spine' appearance in AS.

(a)

(b)

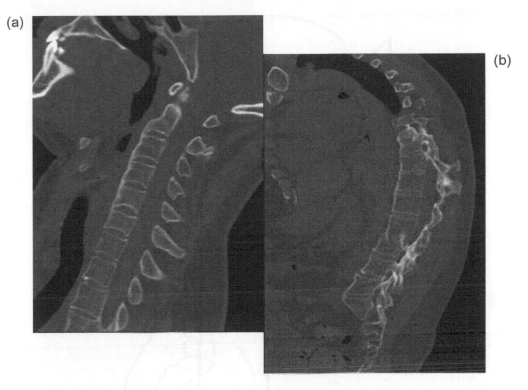

Figure 32.4 Sagittal slice of cervical spine CT scan showing (a) joint ankylosis and (b) loss of lumbar lordosis with fusion and kyphotic deformity centred at the L2/3 level.

Q: What are the systemic manifestations of this condition?

AS is related to a series of autoimmune diseases, including inflammatory bowel disease, anterior uveitis and psoriasis. Systemic manifestations include acute anterior uveitis and iritis, heart disease (cardiac conduction abnormalities), pulmonary fibrosis, renal amyloidosis and ascending aortic conditions such as aortitis, stenosis, regurgitation. *Klebsilella pneumoniae* synovitis is a rare condition that is more commonly seen in HLA-B27 positive individuals.

Q: What is the systemic treatment for this condition, and how can the deformity be managed?

The mainstays of pharmacological treatment in AS are NSAIDs and TNF-α inhibitors (TNFis). Additional treatments include non-TNFi biologic medications, methotrexate and sulfasalazine. Local injections of glucocorticoids are effective in treating enthesopathy and arthritis.

Correction of spinal deformity in AS is complex and relies on thorough preoperative planning. Relevant factors include the location of the apex of the curve and its flexibility. This can be assessed by flexion and extension plain radiographs. Relevant radiographic measures include the chin–brow vertical angle (CBVA) and C7 plumb line (Figure 32.5), pelvic incidence (PI) and lumbar lordosis (LL; Figure 32.2).

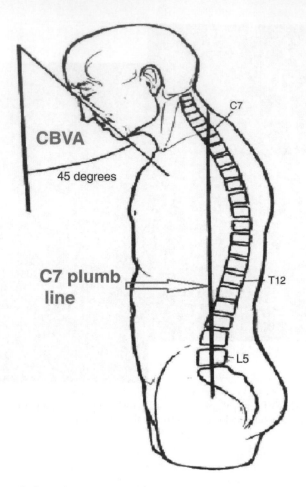

Figure 32.5 Relevant radiological parameters in AS.

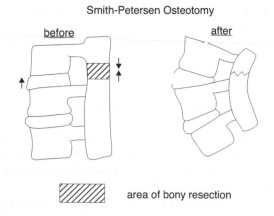

Figure 32.6 Area of bony resection in Smith-Petersen osteotomy.

Spinal deformity can be surgically corrected by a combination of soft tissue released and osteotomies (bony cuts). The two most described are the Smith–Petersen osteotomy (SPO) and the pedicle subtracting osteotomy (PSO; See spinal osteotomy q. 30; Figure 32.6).

Before   after

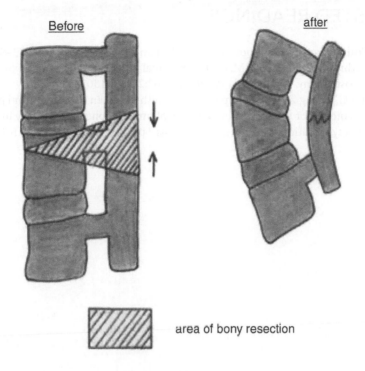

area of bony resection

Figure 32.7   Area of bony resection in Pedicle subtraction osteotomy.

The PSO is a more powerful osteotomy where body cuts through the pedicle (trans-pedicular) and into vertebral body are used to correct deformity (Figure 32.7).

The location of the osteotomy is determined by the nature of the deformity. Cervico-thoracic kyphosis (chin-on-chest deformity) can be managed by **C7–T1 cervico-thoracic osteotomy, while thoracolumbar kyphosis can be managed by osteotomies in the lumbar spine.** Management of spinal deformity in patients with coexisting hip arthritis should be managed in discussion with the arthroplasty surgeons so that a decision can be made about which pathology should be managed first. In many cases, the spinal deformity is corrected first so that version of the acetabular and femoral components can be calculated from a stable spinal position.

Exam Tips

- Neutral balance = C7 plumb line passing within 2cm of the posterosuperior corner of the S1 vertebral body on lateral X-ray (XR) of the lumbar spine.
- The exact aetiology of AS remains unclear, but a close correlation between AS and the HLA (human leukocyte antigen) B27 has been observed.
- Detailed understanding of the technical steps to perform various osteotomy types is beyond the expected scope of the FRCS exam. You should be able to describe the two main osteotomies in general terms, however!
- Remember the key differences between DISH and AS. These patients are stable, with clear examinations findings, and so these topics are frequently examined.

SUGGESTED READINGS

1. Sieper J, Poddubnyy D. Axial spondyloarthritis. Lancet. 2017;390(10089):73–84.
2. Ahn UM, Ahn NU, Buchowski JM, et al. Functional outcome and radiographic correction after spinal osteotomy. Spine (Phila Pa 1976). 2002;27(12):1303–11.
3. Liu H, Yang C, Zheng Z, et al. Comparison of Smith-Petersen osteotomy and pedicle subtraction osteotomy for the correction of thoracolumbar kyphotic deformity in ankylosing spondylitis: a systematic review and meta-analysis. Spine (Phila Pa 1976). 2015;40(8):570–9.

SECTION 5
PRIMARY TUMOURS

33

OSTEOID OSTEOMA

You are referred a 20-year-old male with 6 months of persistent thoracic back pain without a history of trauma. The pain is worst at night and on drinking alcohol. He has been managing this with oral aspirin. He denies weight loss, bowel, or bladder symptoms. He has no other medical history.

On examination, he has tenderness on palpation over the mid-thoracic spine. He is neurologically intact in both upper and lower limbs. The referring doctor requested a plain radiograph of the thoracic spine (not shown), which did not give a definitive diagnosis due to poor visualisation. A CT scan of the thoracic spine was performed (Figure 33.1).

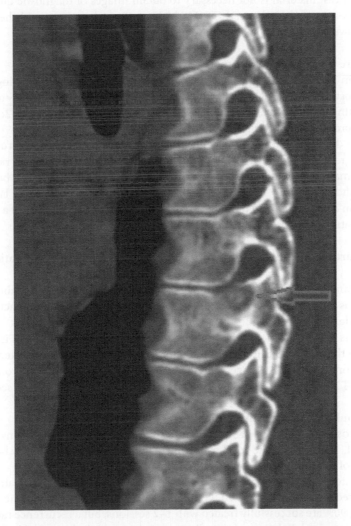

Figure 33.1 Sagittal CT shows a focal lytic lesion (nidus) with central density, suspicious of calcification in the right T8 pedicle, with very minimal sclerotic reaction seen surrounding the nidus.

DOI: 10.1201/9781003201304-38

Q: What is the working diagnosis?

The symptoms and imaging are suggestive of osteoid osteoma. Osteoid osteoma accounts for 13.5% of all benign tumours. Most of those affected are young; approximately one-half are in the 2nd decade of life at presentation. The most common symptom is bone pain, which often worsens at night. The pain is thought to be mediated by release of prostaglandins, which helps explain the relief experienced after prostaglandin inhibitors such as NSAIDs such as aspirin.

Spinal lesions account for 10% of osteoid osteomas. The lesions involve the lumbar, cervical and thoracic spinal segments, in order of decreasing frequency. Involvement of the posterior elements is more common than that of the vertebral body. The spinal canal and paraspinous soft tissues are not affected.

CT remains the modality of choice for detecting osteoid osteoma and generally provides the best characterisation of both the nidus and the surrounding cortical sclerosis. The nidus appears as a well-defined radiolucent region and demonstrates varying degrees of central mineralisation in approximately 50% of cases. Although the use of intravenous contrast material is not necessary to obtain images of diagnostic quality, the nidus enhances at contrast-enhanced CT. Marked reactive sclerosis around the nidus is common; however, some lesions may have little to no reactive sclerosis.

Q: What are the differential diagnoses of this condition?

The main differential diagnosis is osteoblastoma, which may be indistinguishable from osteoid osteoma at radiologic imaging. The lesion size and natural history are its main differentiating features: Osteoblastoma tends to be larger (nidus diameter >2cm) and exhibit growth progression on serial imaging.

Other differential diagnoses include a Brodie abscess (may resemble an osteoid osteoma at radiography, CT and MRI), stress fracture (also has osteosclerosis at radiography and CT and marrow oedema at MRI; however, no nidus is seen), aneurysmal bone cyst (ABC) and chondroblastoma. The lytic focus in chondroblastoma tends to be larger and more lobular in contour than the nidus of osteoid osteoma, and the presence of a calcified chondroid matrix is suggestive of the diagnosis.

Q: What further imaging could you request, and what do these investigations classically show?

Bone scan may be useful for lesion location. It shows intense metabolic activity of the nidus and relatively decreased activity in the surrounding reactive zone—the double-density sign.

MRI is not always necessary but can add additional information (Figure 33.2). The signal in the nidus typically is isointense to that of muscle on T1-weighted images and is variable on T2-weighted images. Signal hyperintensity is seen in the surrounding reactive zone on T2-weighted or short inversion time inversion recovery (STIR) sequences.

Q: How would you manage this patient?

Osteoid osteoma may be self-limiting, and the regression of some lesions has been documented. NSAIDs provide good pain control, but its long-term use may be unacceptable because of refractory pain or gastrointestinal complications.

CT guided radiofrequency ablation is the current gold standard of treatment. This uses a radiofrequency probe at 80–90 °C for 6 minutes to produce a 1cm zone of necrosis. Of patients, 90% are successfully treated with 1–2 sessions, but a recurrence rate of up to 15% has been reported. Relative contraindications to its use include a spinal lesion located near neural tissue.

(a)

(b)

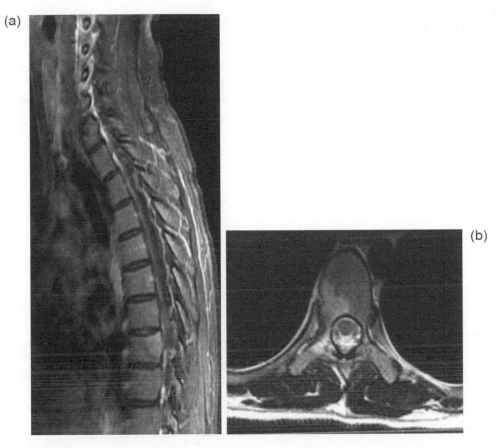

Figure 33.2 MRI scan thoracic spine (a) sagittal (T1-weighted) and (b) axial (T2-weighted, T8 level) showing a focal area of hypo-intensity in the posterior aspect of the right side of T8 vertebral body with involvement of the right pedicle.

Complete surgical resection with curettage of the nidus has historically been the treatment of choice for osteoid osteoma and can be performed open or percutaneously. Resection leaves a bone defect that may be vulnerable to fracture and, in some cases, may necessitate internal fixation and bone grafting. It is indicated where the location of the lesion does not allow radiofrequency ablation or in spinal lesions with associated scoliosis. The associated scoliosis rarely requires treatment.

Exam Tips

- Osteoid osteoma is a small, benign but painful lesion with specific clinical and imaging characteristics. Classical X-ray findings are of a circular cortical lucency representing the nidus (usually less than 1.5cm in diameter) with surrounding sclerosis.
- X-ray is rarely diagnostic of osteoid osteoma.
- The main differential diagnosis is osteoblastoma and you should be aware of the key radiological differences between the two. CT scan is the preferred imaging modality.
- Always think of an osteoid osteoma when faced with a case of painful scoliosis in the adolescent population.

SUGGESTED READINGS

1.   Mallepally AR, Mahajan R, Pacha S, et al. Spinal osteoid osteoma: Surgical resection and review of literature. Surg Neurol Int. 2020;11:308.
2.   Chai JW, Hong SH, Choi JY, et al. Radiologic diagnosis of osteoid osteoma: from simple to challenging findings. Radiographics. 2010;30(3):737–49.

34

SCHWANNOMA

Q: A 71-year-old-female presents to the outpatient clinic complaining of a 1-year history of progressive left arm numbness and hand weakness. She has moderate radicular pain in the arm. In the past few months, she has also noted progressive weakness and stiffness in her leg and now walks with a cane. **How do you proceed?**

The history is suggestive of pathology in the cervical spine causing the left arm symptoms and what may represent myelopathy. My differential at this stage is broad and I would therefore like to elicit more from the history and learn about the presence of any red flags, for example systemic symptoms or weight loss. I would like to perform a full neurological examination of the patient and arrange an MRI scan.

Q: The scan is shown below. Please comment on how you would proceed?

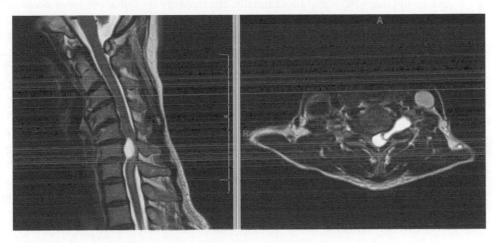

The scans show an intradural extramedullary lesion centred in the left C6/7 foramen. The cord is compressed and displaced, and there is complete effacement of the CSF. There is abnormal signal within the cord which may represent myelomalacia. The lesion appears dumbbell-shaped, and my first differential would be a nerve sheath tumour. Other differential diagnoses include meningioma and neurofibroma.

Q: **Examination reveals a wide-based, unsteady gait. Romberg test is positive. Lower extremity reflexes are brisk. In her left upper extremity, power is reduced Medical Research Council (MRC) grade 4/5 in C7, C8 and 2/5 in T1. What would be your next steps?**

This patient is presenting with a combination of myelopathy and left radicular symptoms with weakness. There is cord compression evident on the scan and in combination with the progressive deficit that necessitates prompt surgical decompression. I would discuss this case with the nearest tertiary neurosurgical unit as it requires specialist neurosurgical care.

Q: What surgery do you think will need to be performed, and what are the main risks you would foresee?

I would anticipate a multilevel laminectomy, attempted gross total resection of the lesion and posterior instrumentation. Intra-operative monitoring, including motor and sensory evoked potentials, would need to be employed to improve the safety profile. I would counsel the patient regarding the risks of paralysis/serious neurological injury, peripheral nerve palsy, cerebrospinal fluid (CSF) leak, infection, bleeding, hardware failure, medical and anaesthetic risks and recurrence. I would counsel the patients that while some recovery is possible, complete recovery is unlikely and will most likely require a period of inpatient rehabilitation.

Q: The patient undergoes a C5–C7 laminectomy, intradural tumour resection and posterior instrumented fixation. Histological analysis of the specimen shows it to be a schwannoma. What do you know about this pathology and what is the likely prognosis or this patient?

Spinal schwannomas are slow growing benign lesions that derive from Schwann cells and may occur throughout the spine and arise from a single nerve fascicle. Most are intradural lesions but may extend extra-foraminally. The majority are solitary but may occur as multiple lesions and are an important pathological feature of neurofibromatosis type 2. The treatment is gross total resection and when this achieved the prognosis is very good, with recurrence rates quoted in the literature of between 5–10%.

Exam Tips

- Schwannomas represent about 25% of all spinal tumours and knowledge of their key features and differential diagnosis as listed above is important. It is also important to recognise that these cases need to be referred to a neurosurgical unit for definitive management.
- Although these tumours are benign, they can cause significant local and radicular pain and myelopathic features, and such cases require prompt surgical resection. Asymptomatic cases that are stable in size may be monitored with regular outpatient follow-up.
- Whilst schwannoma should alert the candidate to the possibility of NF2, NF1 is also a favourite topic in the FRCS exam. Typically, cases tend to be centred on diagnostic criteria or management of scoliosis in NF1.

REFERENCE

Kalra RR, Gottfried ON, Schmidt MH. Spinal schwannomas: an updated review of surgical approaches. Contemp Neurosurg. 2015;37(15):1–8.

35

CERVICAL CHORDOMA

Q: A 49-year-old- male presents to your clinic complaining of a 6-month history of progressively worsening left-sided neck pain and sporadic sinusitis. He has recently noticed some occasional difficulty swallowing but no difficulty breathing. He was seen in the ENT outpatient clinic and a CT and subsequently an MRI scan was arranged, as shown. **Can you comment?**

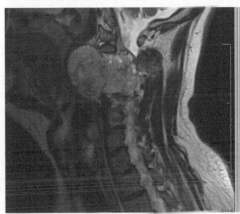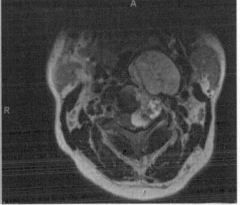

This shows a T2-weighted sagittal and axial MRI. MRI demonstrates a large mass which enhances on T2 imaging. It appears to be in contact with the spinal cord. It also appears to be exerting a mass effect on the oropharyngeal airway. My differential diagnosis based on this imaging would include chondrosarcoma, chordoma, giant cell tumour, plasmacytoma or solitary metastasis. In the first instance, I would like to assess the patient clinically. My primary concern is that this is a primary bone tumour, and given the rarity and complexity of these cases, I would therefore like to discuss this with a tertiary/quaternary specialist unit that offers specialist care in these cases.

Q: Assuming you are the local specialist centre, how do you proceed?
I would like to arrange further systemic staging imaging in the form of CT chest abdomen and pelvis and a whole-spine MRI. I would also like a positron emission tomography (PET) CT and bone scan. Following this I would also like to arrange a CT-guided biopsy. This needs to be carefully planned with the radiologist and with involvement of the treating surgeon to ensure the biopsy tract is excised within the surgical specimen.

Q: CT biopsy demonstrates this is a chordoma. How do you proceed with management?
Chordoma is an uncommon primary tumour that is aggressive and locally invasive and has a poor prognosis. Given that this is a primary tumour, it should be treated in a specialist centre by a surgical team with appropriate expertise as suggested.

Q: Are you aware of any staging systems for this condition?

The principles of the Enneking staging system, originally described for appendicular tumours, apply. Tumours are described as benign or malignant; benign lesions as latent, active or aggressive. Malignant lesions are classified according to grade (low vs high), local extension and the presence of metastasis. In 1997 the Weinstein–Boriani–Biagini (WBB) surgical staging system was presented to standardise terminology and staging of bone tumours, expanding on the Enneking system, and to aid in surgical planning. This system divides the spine into 12 equal zones—numbered in clockwise order—and 5 layers from superficial to deep. En bloc excision is defined in Weinstein et al. (1997) as removal of tumour in one piece with a margin of healthy tissue. Marginal resection involves a surgical plane passing through the pseudocapsule and/or the reactive tissue surrounding the tumour. Intralesional resection refers to cases in which the tumour mass has been breached by the surgeon.

Q: How do you think this patient should be managed?

Summary recommendations from Focus Issues in Spine Oncology for Primary Bone Tumours in 2009 recommend optimal management for chordoma (and chondrosarcoma) is en-bloc resection with wide or marginal margins. Adjuvant radiotherapy of at least 60 to 65 Gy equivalents is also indicated when there is incomplete resection or an intralesional margin.

Q: What are the challenges in performing en bloc resection in this patient?

A previous systematic review by the Spine Oncology Study Group in 2009 showed en bloc resection to be associated with significantly improved continuous disease-free survival and demonstrated open biopsy and intralesional resection to be associated with decreased disease-free survival. However, it also showed a high rate of morbidity both planned, for example nerve root sacrifice, and unplanned, for example local recurrence. This case would therefore require extensive planning and a thorough decision-making process with the patient.

The procedure would need to involve a posterior and then anterior procedure and then possibly a return to the back to insert instrumentation. Sacrifice of nerve roots at this level may have a deleterious effect on diaphragmatic function. The imaging suggests that the vertebral artery is included on the left side and may need to be sacrificed and thorough assessment of the contralateral artery would need to be undertaken. Following surgery, the patient would need to stay in intensive care unit (ICU) and may need a trachcostomy.

Following surgery, the specimen needs to be sent for histological description of the margins, and on this basis, it should be decided whether the patient requires adjuvant radiation therapy.

Exam Tips

- The principles of management of primary bone tumours of the spine that will be tested at FRCS level are by far more important than knowing the nuances of each tumour type and the details of surgery in what is still an evolving field. The most important step is recognition that this may be a primary bone tumour and refer to an appropriate specialist centre as failure to do this, and subsequent intralesional resection, may potentially transform a curable lesion into a fatal one.
- Local and systemic staging needs to be undertaken with the investigations as outlined above. A well-planned biopsy should then be sought and should be performed by the centre that will treat the tumour with involvement of the treating surgeon.

- En bloc resection with wide or marginal margins should be undertaken for surgical treatment of primary malignant bone tumours (2009 Spine Oncology Study Group recommendation).
- Neoadjuvant chemotherapy is recommended in Ewing's sarcoma and osteosarcoma. Adjuvant high-dose radiotherapy is recommended in chordoma and chondrosarcoma when resection is incomplete/intralesional (both are radioresistant).
- Primary malignant tumours include chordoma, chondrosarcoma, osteosarcoma and Ewing's sarcoma. Benign aggressive lesions include aneurysmal bone cyst, giant cell tumour and osteoblastoma.
- The earlier mentioned forms the mainstay of management of these tumours and will achieve a good score in the FRCS exam; nonetheless, an appreciation that other treatment modalities exist is useful. Medical oncology may prescribe denosumab in neo-adjuvant treatment of GCT to reduce tumour size and improve pain. Interventional radiology performs procedures such as selective arterial embolisation in ABC, and thermal ablation in osteoid osteoma.
- Spine stereotactic body radiotherapy (SBRT) can deliver high doses of radiation to a focused area whilst sparing at-risk tissue and, although traditionally used for metastatic disease, is also being used in primary tumours. Proton therapy limits dosage to surrounding tissue and is used in primary tumours. Carbon–ion therapy is an evolving therapy with promising local control rates.

SUGGESTED READINGS

1. Boriani S, Weinstein JN, Biagini R, et al. Spine Update. Primary bone tumours of the spine: terminology and surgical staging. Spine. 1997;22(9):1036–44.
2. Yamazaki T, McLoughlin GS, Patel S, et al. Feasibility and safety of en bloc resection for primary spine tumours: a systematic review by the Spine Oncology Study Group. Spine. 2009;34:S31–8.
3. Charest-Morin R, Fisher CG, Sahgal A, et al. Primary bone tumours of the spine—an evolving field: what the general spine surgeon should know. Global Spine J. 2019;9(1 Suppl):108S–16S.

SECTION 6
METASTATIC SPINAL TUMOURS

36

RENAL METASTASIS

A 64-year-old male is referred from the ED to the on-call orthopaedic team. He has a known history of renal cell carcinoma treated in the previous year with partial nephrectomy. He smokes 10 cigarettes per day and has lost around 7 kg in weight over the previous 3 months.

He complains of significant lower back pain, worsened by ambulation and at night, with shooting pain into the anterior aspect of his right thigh. On examination, he has no upper motor neurone signs but has weakness of hip flexion bilaterally (Grade 3) and reduced sensation along his right groin crease and upper thigh. He reports normal bowel and bladder function.

Q: Which initial investigations should be performed, and what is the working diagnosis?

Given the patient's history and age, I would like to exclude a diagnosis of a metastatic spinal deposit. After completion of a detailed neurological exam, I would ensure that the patient had a staging CT chest, abdomen and pelvis as well as baseline bloods, including full blood count with differential, erythrocyte sedimentation rate basic metabolic panel, serum and urine immune-electrophoresis (SPEP, UPEP, respectively) and tumour markers.

I would obtain an MRI scan of the whole spine to exclude malignant deposits which could be a cause of his back and anterior thigh pain. A technetium bone scan could further identify the extent of disease.

It is essential to measure blood calcium as malignant hypercalcaemia can be a medical emergency associated with metastatic bone disease. (Symptoms include confusion, muscle weakness, nausea and polydipsia/polyuria). In a patient where a spinal lesion was seen, without the identification of a primary tumour, a CT-guided biopsy would be necessary to rule out a primary bone lesion.

The staging CT scan revealed a recurrence mass in the patient's right kidney. This was confirmed to be a renal cell carcinoma.

MRI and CT scans of the lumbar spine are shown in Figures 36.1 and 36.2, respectively.

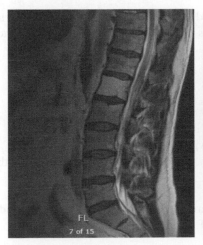 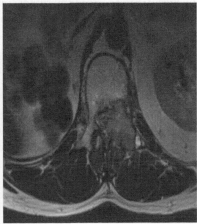

Figure 36.1   MRI scan (T2-weighted) lateral and axial (L1) showing spinal lesion.

DOI: 10.1201/9781003201304-42

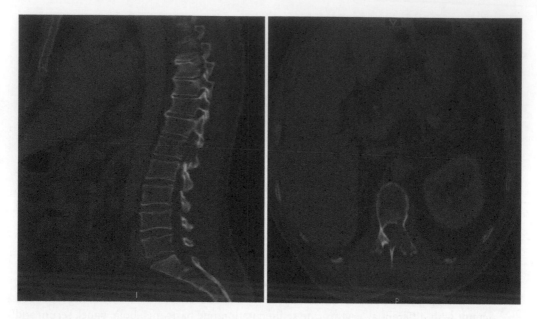

Figure 36.2 CT scan lateral and axial (L1) showing lytic lesion with involvement of L1 pedicle, lamina and spinous process.

Q: What is the cause of the spinal symptoms in this patient, and how can this patient be classified?

These images show a left-sided metastatic renal deposit to the L1 vertebra causing dural compression. The tumour involves the posterior elements and L1 foramen.

Renal cell cancer (RCC) is known to be highly vascular and relatively radioresistant. Bone metastases are one of the most common metastatic sites and occur in around 30% of RCCs. Patients with metastatic deposits in spine can be classified according to the spinal instability neoplastic score (SINS). Patients who are classified as unstable or potentially unstable can be surgically stabilised by either percutaneous or open approaches (Table 36.1).

The Bilsky (ESCC—epidural spinal cord compression) grading evaluates the severity of spinal cord compression on cross sections obtained with T2-weighted MRI and can also be used (Figure 36.3):

- Low Grade
  - 0: bone disease alone
  - 1: epidural impingement
  - 1a: epidural impingement without deformation of the thecal sac
  - 1b: deformation of the thecal sac without spinal cord abutment
  - 1c: deformation of the thecal sac with spinal cord abutment but without cord compression
- High Grade
  - 2: spinal cord compression with cerebrospinal fluid (CSF) visible around the cord
  - 3: spinal cord compression, no CSF visible around the cord

Table 36.1 Spinal instability neoplastic score

	Score
Spine Location	
Junctional (occiput-C2, C7-T2, TII-LI, L5-S1)	3
Mobile spine (C3-6, L2-4)	2
Semi-rigid (T3-10)	1
Rigid (S2-5)	0
Mechanical or postural pain	
Yes	3
No (occasional pain but not mechanical)	1
Pain-free lesion	0
Bone lesion quality	
Lytic	2
Mixed lytic/blastic	1
Blastic	0
Radiographic spinal alignment	
Subluxation/translation present	4
De novo deformity (kyphosis/scoliosis)	2
Normal alignment	0
Vertebral body involvement	
>50% collapse	3
<50% collapse	2
No collapse with >50% of the body involved	1
None of the above	0
Posterior involvement	
Bilateral	3
Unilateral	1
None of the above	0

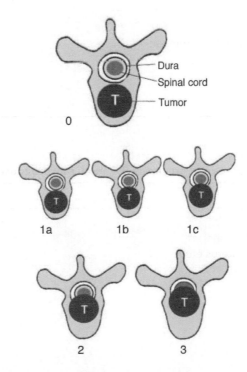

Figure 36.3   Schematic representation of the six-point Bilsky ESCC grading scale.

Several prognostic scoring systems exist. These include the *Tomita score*, which is composed of 3 parameters based on tumour growth, visceral metastases and number of bone metastasis lesions (Table 36.3).

Another is the modified Tokuhashi prognostic score, based on 6 elements: general condition, extraspinal bony metastasis, number of vertebral bodies with metastasis, visceral metastasis, primary tumour and neurologic compromise (Table 36.2).

Table 36.2 Modified Tokuhashi score (>11 good prognosis, 9–11 moderate prognosis, <8 poor prognosis)

Prognosis parameter	Score
Patient condition	
Poor (performance status 10-40%)	0
Moderate (performance status 50-70%)	1
Good (performance status 80-100%)	2
No. of bone metastases outside spine	
>2	0
1-2	1
0	2
Mets. to major organs	
Non-removable	0
Removable	1
None	2
Primary site	
Lung, osteosarcoma, stomach, bladder, oesophagus, pancreas	0
Liver, gallbladder, unidentified	1
Other	2
Kidney, uterus	3
Rectum	4
Thyroid, breast, prostate, carcinoid tumour	5
Palsy	
Complete (Frankel A,B)	0
Incomplete (Frankel C,D)	1
None (Frankel E)	2

Table 36.3 Tomita score (2–4 good prognosis, 5–7 moderate prognosis, 8–10 poor prognosis)

Prognosis parameter	Score
Primary site	
Slow growth (breast, thyroid, etc)	1
Moderate growth (kidney, uterus etc)	2
Rapid growth (lung, stomach etc)	4
Visceral metastases	
None	0
Treatable	2
Not treatable	4
Bone Metastases	
Solitary	1
Multiple	2

Q: How should this patient be managed?

I would ensure that the patient was managed in a multidisciplinary manner along with the oncology and pain team. A spinal lesion represents a distant metastasis in RCC; therefore, these patients are stage IV and treatment considerations should include life expectancy, the burden of systemic disease, mechanical stability, degree of myelopathy and presence of pain or other neurological symptoms.

The goals of treatment should focus on pain palliation, local tumour control, mechanical stability and neurologic protection/restoration.

Treatment of spinal metastases in RCC is based on surgery, radiotherapy and systemic therapy. This patient has evidence of neurological compression from a traditionally radioresistant tumour and will likely require surgical management in conjunction with post-operative radiotherapy.

The Patchell et al. paper was a randomised, multicentre non-blinded trial published in the *Lancet* in 2005. It randomly assigned patients with spinal cord compression caused by metastatic cancer to either surgery followed by radiotherapy (n=50) or radiotherapy alone (n=51). The study found that direct decompressive surgery plus post-operative radiotherapy is superior to treatment with radiotherapy alone for patients with spinal cord compression caused by metastatic cancer.

Traditionally, RCC is reported to be radioresistant to conventional fractionated external radiotherapy (RT). Concerns about high radiation dose and the lack of effective targeting with traditional radiotherapy techniques have led to the increased use of stereotactic beam radiotherapy. They consist of delivering a high dose, in 1–3 fractions, into a small target, with rapid 'fall-off' of the dose, enabling the radiation dose to be confined more precisely to treatment volume while sparing the spinal cord or other critical structures.

Stereotactic-radiosurgery (SRS; 1 fraction) or SBRT (2–3 fractions) have been developed. These techniques require a precise location of the tumour. SBRT, using T1 and T2 axial MRI scans fused with CT scans to localise the tumour, has been shown to be effective with durable local control, progression-free survival and palliation rates of approximately 70–90% in patients receiving de novo treatment.

Spinal metastases from RCC are known to be highly vascular at risk of significant intra-operative blood loss and post-operative haematomas. Arterial embolisation (the injection of coils, liquid or particle agents directly into the feeding artery of the tumour) should be performed before any surgery is attempted.

A diagnostic spinal angiography should be carried out before embolisation with 2 objectives: first, to assess vascularisation of the lesion and, second, to determine whether an anterior spinal artery shares the same pedicle as the feeding artery of the tumour. Surgery should be performed within 24–48h after embolisation to avoid revascularisation of the tumour by collateral vessels.

The aim for surgery is to control pain, maintain ambulation, continence, muscle strength and functional ability. The surgical approach depends on the tumour location. The traditional approach in this case would be laminectomy and posterior stabilisation, followed by post-operative RT.

Separation surgery is a more novel concept in which the aim is to establish a margin of a few millimetres between the tumour and the spinal cord/dural sac. This facilitates the most effective targeting of post-operative SBRT while minimising the risk of damage to neural structures. SBRT is associated with a risk of vertebral compression fracture. Other complications of surgery followed by SBRT treatment include wound breakdown or dehiscence, although this risk is lower than following conventional external beam RT.

Exam Tips

- General considerations in the management of metastatic lesions to the spine can be summarised by the NOMS framework—neurological, oncologic, mechanical stability and systemic illness.
- Remember the importance of an overall consideration of the patient's medical status. Patients in a metastatic setting are likely to have decreased performance status and to be fragile.
- Detailed descriptions of the pros and cons of the various surgical approaches isn't particularly necessary. In reality, this will depend on the location of the lesion. For most metastatic lesions to the spine, particularly in a patient with clear neurological symptoms and cord compression, you certainly won't be marked down for describing a posterior decompression (laminectomy) at the level of compression and post-operative radiotherapy. However, in the setting of renal metastasis, given its radio resistence, an awareness of the advent of SBRT and separation surgery will ensure that you score well.
- The Patchell et al. paper (see the References) is a seminal paper in the understanding of metastatic cord compression. Essential reading before the exam!

SUGGESTED READINGS

1. Patchell RA, Tibbs PA, Regine WF, et al. Direct decompressive surgical resection in the treatment of spinal cord compression caused by metastatic cancer: a randomised trial. Lancet. 2005;366:643–8.
2. Teyssonneau D, Gross-Goupil M, Domblides C, et al. Treatment of spinal metastases in renal cell carcinoma: a critical review. Crit Rev Oncol Hematol. 2018;125:19–29.
3. Goodwin C, Karim A, Boone C. The challenges of renal cell carcinoma metastatic to the spine: a systematic review of survival and treatment. Global Spine J. 2018;8(5):517–26.
4. Thibault I, Al-Omair A, Masucci GL, et al. Spine stereotactic body radiotherapy for renal cell cancer spinal metastases: analysis of outcomes and risk of vertebral compression fracture. J Neurosurg Spine. 2014;21(5):711–18.

37

MYELOMA

An 80-year-old male referred to the orthopaedic team from the ED. He complains of sudden weakness in both legs over the preceding 48h, with severe pain in the thoracic spine, worsened by movement. He has lost around 6 kg of weight over the previous 2 months.

On examination, he has brisk patella and ankle reflexes and lower limb hypertonia. Upper limb power and sensation is symmetrically normal. He has Medical Research Council (MRC) grade 2 power on hip and knee flexion/extension. He was ataxic with an inability to heel–toe walk.

X-ray, MRI scan (Figure 37.1) and CT scan (Figure 37.2) of the whole spine are performed.

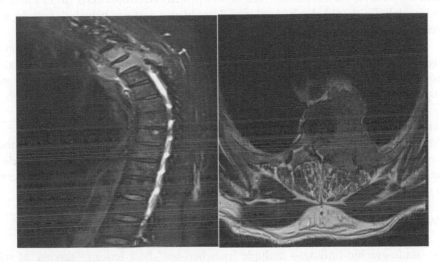

Figure 37.1 MRI thoracic spine (T2-weighted) lateral and axial (T2/T3) showing large paraspinous mass with soft tissue component and extension into the spinal canal.

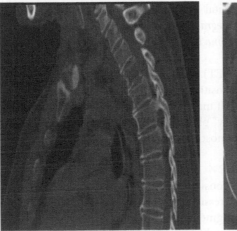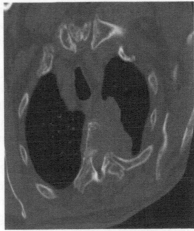

Figure 37.2 CT scan thoracic spine showing lytic lesion of the T3 vertebral body with involvement of posterior elements.

DOI: 10.1201/9781003201304-43

Q: What do these images show?

The spinal lesion is poorly visualised on X-ray. The MRI scan shows a large T2/3 par-aspinal mass with thecal sac compression. *(Note: Additional smaller lesions were seen at T12 and within the left clavicle.)* Osseous lysis is seen in the T3 vertebral body, pedicle, left transverse process, lamina and posterior rib. There is intraspinal extension into the epidural space with compression of the thecal sac.

Q: What is the diagnosis?

Differential diagnoses include multiple osseous metastases, myeloma and lymphoma.

Q: What investigations would you perform?

I would order a staging CT chest abdomen and pelvis to exclude a metastatic deposit. I would request blood tests, including full blood count, urea and creatinine, calcium and erythrocyte sedimentation rate. Serum protein electrophoresis (SPEP) and beta-2-microglobulin should also be requested. I would also perform urinalysis looking for proteinuria. Urine protein electrophoresis may show Bence Jones proteins.

Definitive diagnosis is via CT guided biopsy. The percentage of plasma cells on histology is the major criteria used to distinguish plasmacytoma (10–30% plasma cells) versus multiple myeloma (>30% plasma cells) *(*normal amount of plasma cells on bone marrow aspirate is <2%).*

Q: How common is multiple myeloma, and how can it be classified?

Multiple myeloma is the second-most common haematological malignancy and the most common malignancy involving bone. The spine is the most frequently affected skeletal site in multiple myeloma. Spinal cord or cauda equina compression is reported to develop in 11–24% of myeloma patients with myeloma spinal disease.

Q: What are the classical radiological findings of multiple myeloma?

- Radiographic findings—multiple "punched-out" lytic lesions (absence of sclerotic border results from the lack of osteoblastic activity)—only visible once >50% destruction has occurred.
- MRI—dark on T1- and bright on T2-weighted image.
- Bone scan—Cold in 30% so skeletal survey is recommended. *('Hot' areas on bone scan are caused by radio-tracer integration into the inorganic phase of bone caused by osteoblastic activity. Multiple myeloma bone scans are cold due to the lack of osteoblastic activity.)*
- Positron emission tomography (PET) scans—fluorodeoxyglucose-positron emission tomography (FDG-PET)—93% sensitivity and more sensitive than plain radiographs in diagnosing/screening for MM. It may uncover additional previously unrecognised sites in wrongly diagnosed "solitary" plasmacytoma. Uptake into cancer cells is due to increased glucose metabolism in most types of tumours.

Q: How would you manage this patient?

A multidisciplinary approach should consider systemic chemotherapy, pain control, relief of spinal cord or cauda equina compression and maintenance of spinal stability. Additional interventions such as cement augmentation, radiotherapy or surgery are often necessary to prevent, treat and control spinal complications.

Stability can be assessed using the SINS. Overt spinal instability can lead to neurological impairment and severe pain. Cement augmentation is considered for patients with vertebral compression fractures for pain control and to increase the strength and stiffness of the vertebral body. The 2019 guidelines from the International Myeloma Working Group (IMWG) recommend that all newly diagnosed symptomatic myeloma patients receive bisphosphonate treatment. The aim of bisphosphonate treatment is to slow down or prevent the progression of bone destruction and, in the process, can help alleviate bone pain and reduce the risk of skeletal fractures. Zoledronic acid is currently the preferred choice as it is also associated with improved survival.

Anti-Myeloma Treatment

Current anti-myeloma regimens combine chemotherapy agents with steroids and either proteasome inhibitors or immunomodulatory drugs, with or without high-dose chemotherapy and stem cell transplantation. High-dose steroids can reduce swelling and inflammation and provide rapid pain control and improvement, particularly in cases involving spinal cord compression.

RT

Myeloma lesions are extraordinarily radiosensitive and for patients with levels of spinal pain that significantly affect day-to-day function, RT can be useful for its control. Several studies have demonstrated its efficacy in alleviating pain and maintaining mobility in patients. RT is also indicated for the treatment of epidural or extramedullary masses at risk of, or causing, spinal cord or cauda equina compression.

Spinal Treatment

Bracing—This procedure may provide short-term control of pain by stabilising the spine and reducing the mechanical load on the vertebral bodies.

Surgery—Safe instrumentation can be extremely challenging due to the weakness of the vertebra due to infiltration. **In most cases, epidural tumours are treated very effectively by steroids/chemotherapy and RT, without the need for surgical decompression.** Surgical intervention is reserved for those with significant spinal instability, for example where there has been significant destruction to all three bony columns of the spine (SINS score).

Vertebral augmentation—There is increasing evidence that kyphoplasty (the insertion of cement into the vertebral body after the use of a vertebral balloon to create a cavity within the infiltrated bone) can improve pain and stability.

Exam Tips

- This is a frequently examined topic so you should know it in depth. Be aware of the lab findings (both serum and urinalysis). Remember 'CRAB' as a useful memory aid: hyperCalcaemia, Renal Failure, Anaemia, Bone lesions.
- Remember that while metastatic deposits may be radioresistant, multiple myeloma is exquisitely radiosensitive and so should be managed by cEBRT (conventional external beam radiotherapy), rather than conventional surgery, in almost all cases in the first instance.

SUGGESTED READINGS

1. Molloy S, Lai M, Pratt G, et al. Optimizing the management of patients with spinal myeloma disease. Br J Haematol. 2015;171:332–43.

2.   Patchell RA, Tibbs PA, Regine WF, et al. Direct decompressive surgical resection treatment of spinal cord compression caused by metastatic cancer: a randomised trial. Lancet. 2005;366:643–8.

3.   Kyriakou C, Molloy S, Vrionis F, et al. The role of cement augmentation with percutaneous vertebroplasty and balloon kyphoplasty for the treatment of vertebral compression fractures in multiple myeloma: a consensus statement from the International Myeloma Working Group (IMWG). Blood Cancer J. 2019;9(3):27.

38

LUNG METASTASIS

Q: A 56-year-old-lady presents with progressive severe neck pain and bilateral arm pain, right worse than left, progressive over the last 3 months. Her CT imaging is shown. Please comment on the CT.

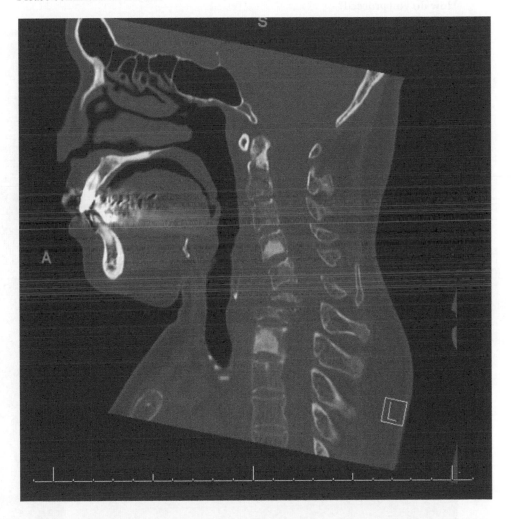

This is a sagittal CT image showing what appear to be multiple mixed blastic and lytic lesions throughout the cervical and upper thoracic spine. There are burst fractures of the C6 and C7 vertebral bodies and a resulting kyphotic deformity. My main differential based on this imaging is metastatic disease, and I would like to learn more about the patient's history. I would also like to perform further investigations to evaluate this patient systemically. Although this CT is only a single sagittal slice, given the kyphosis and history of progressive pain, I would be concerned about stability and imminent risk to the spinal cord. To afford some initial pain relief, I would put the patient into a cervical collar.

DOI: 10.1201/9781003201304-44

Q: On further questioning the patient complains of some compromise to hand function that has developed in the last 6 months. She has developed shortness of breath and weight loss over the same period. Examination reveals a severe restriction in upper limb movement secondary to pain, hyperreflexia and a positive Hoffman's sign. Her gait is unsteady. How do you proceed?

I would like to obtain a CT chest, abdomen and pelvis and a whole-spine MRI scan.

Q: CT chest, abdomen and pelvis demonstrates extensive sclerotic metastatic bony disease and ground glass opacification in the right lung apex. The MRI is shown. How do you proceed?

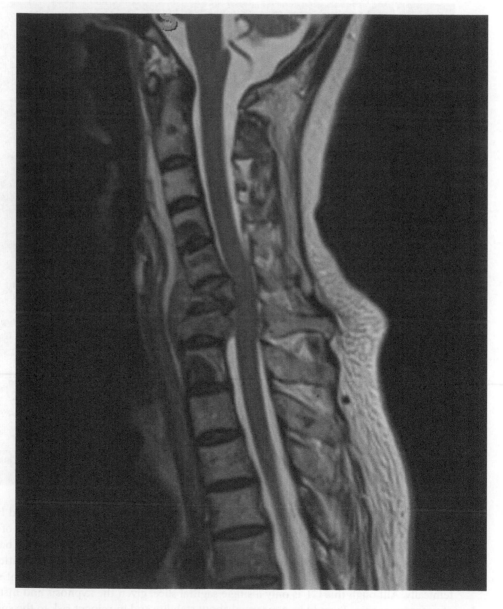

The MRI is suggestive of cord compression which would fit with the myelopathic history and examination findings. The CT chest, abdomen and pelvis results are highly

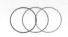

suggestive of metastatic lung cancer. I would start the patient on dexamethasone and a proton pump inhibitor. I would like to obtain tumour markers and contact the oncology service for assessment. I would also calculate a SIN score to further assess her spinal stability.

Q: Can you explain the SIN score?

This is a classification system developed in 2010 by the Spine Oncology Study Group to evaluate spinal instability in the setting of neoplastic disease. Prior to this, spinal instability in this context was highly subjective. The SIN system includes 6 components, each with a weighted value: disease location, pain (mechanical or not), bone lesion (lytic/blastic), spinal alignment, vertebral body collapse and posterolateral element involvement. The maximum score is 18. A score of 0–6 indicates stability, 7–12 is 'indeterminate' and 13–18 indicates instability. This scoring system has been demonstrated in subsequent studies to show good inter- and intra-observer reliability and is thus a useful tool to help guide management.

Q: The SIN score is 15. Following oncological assessment, prognosis is estimated at around 18 months. How would you proceed?

The SIN score is suggestive of instability and is in itself a surgical indication, particularly with the progressive upper limb and neck pain. The development of myelopathy is also a surgical indication. A prognosis of 18 months would be considered good in this setting and appropriate for surgical intervention. Perhaps the most important element of the assessment is however the patient's own wishes, and this would need to be fully addressed with the patient and their family, as they preferred. Multidisciplinary input would be important in this context. The patient would also require an anaesthetic assessment to evaluate fitness for surgery.

Q: The patient decides that they wish to proceed with surgery and are deemed anaesthetically fit. What are the key surgical goals, and can you suggest how this might be achieved?

The goals of surgery in this case would be decompression of the spinal cord and surgical stabilisation. There may be the possibility of decompression of the cervical roots also, depending on where the disease burden lies, and this would need assessing on the pre-operative MRI. This would most likely involve a combined front-and-back procedure, with a 2-level corpectomy (C6, C7), and posterior stabilisation using a long construct, most likely crossing the cervicothoracic junction. Given the likely length of the anterior construct, a longitudinal extensile incision rather than transverse may be helpful.

Exam Tips

- Questions on metastatic disease of the spine should be approached in a systematic way as outlined earlier. The key principles apply regardless of the aetiology of the disease, and so a good score in the FRCS should always be achievable in all such questions.
- Scoring systems: Although details of the different scoring systems used in spine oncology are not required to pass the FRCS exam, knowledge of what they attempt to assess is useful and adds depth to your answers. The NOMS criteria uses neurological, oncological, mechanical (instability), and systemic factors as a framework for decision making in spinal metastatic disease and incorporates the SINS criteria.

- The Tokuhashi Scoring System is a prognostic evaluation system of metastatic spine tumours. It scores 6 criteria, including performance status, no of spinal metastases and presence of neurological palsy (Frankel Grading). The total score recommends either conservative, palliative or excisional surgery. Another similar prognostic scoring system is the Tomita system.

REFERENCE

Fisher CG, DiPaola CP, Ryken TC, et al. A novel classification system for spinal instability in neoplastic disease: an evidence based approach and expert consensus from the Spine Oncology Study Group. Spine. 2010;15(35):E1221–9.

SECTION 7
PAEDIATRIC SPINAL SURGERY

39

ADOLESCENT IDIOPATHIC SCOLIOSIS

A 14-year-old girl presents to a paediatric orthopaedic spinal clinic after her mother noticed a curvature in her back and a prominence of her right shoulder blade. The patient herself reports no pain or dysfunction, but she is concerned about the shape of her shoulders and hips. She is unable to get clothes to fit comfortably, and she believes her shape is progressively worsening.

There is no relevant past medical history. Her mother reports that she has grown in height rapidly over the last 12 months and had her first menstrual period 6 months prior. There is a family history of scoliosis in the maternal grandmother and maternal aunt.

The GP requested a plain radiograph of her whole spine (Figure 39.1) which led to the specialist referral.

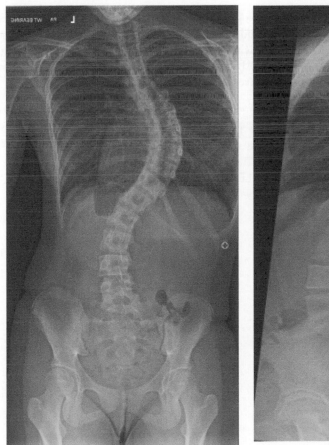
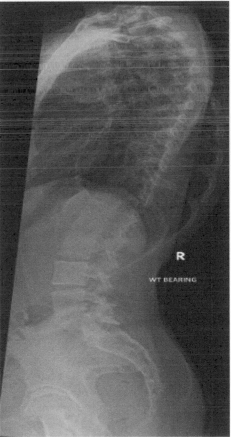

Figure 39.1 Plain radiographs of the whole spine (AP and lateral) showing right-sided thoracic scoliosis with an apex at T8/9.

DOI: 10.1201/9781003201304-46

Q: How would you take a detailed history and examine this patient?

Relevant information includes detailed birth history, developmental milestones, family history of spinal deformity and assessment of physiological maturity (age of menarche).

This patient should be examined in her underwear and bra with a chaperone. General inspection of the child should include comment on body habitus (obesity/underweight) and facial features consistent with underlying conditions such as Down's syndrome.

Other relevant examination findings include the following:

- Shoulder height symmetry
- Presence of truncal shift
- Waist-line asymmetry
- Limb length inequality (LLD; look for shoe lifts or other walking aids. Use measuring blocks to quantify LLD if found)
- Rib prominence
- Café au lait spots (neurofibromatosis)
- Axillary freckles
- Hairy patches or skin dimples on the lower back
- Foot deformities (especially look for cavovarus)

Detailed upper and lower limb neurological examination including abdominal reflexes should be undertaken. (Asymmetrical abdominal reflexes can be a sign of syringomyelia.)

A scoliometer is an instrument that is placed on the back and can be used to provide an objective measure of curve rotation. Always perform a gait assessment (ask the patient to walk while observing from the back, front and side).

Special tests include the following:

- Adams forward bending test (Figure 39.2)
  - Axial plane deformity indicates structural curve.
- Forward bending sitting test
  - This can eliminate the effect of LLD as a cause of the scoliosis.

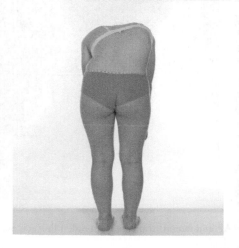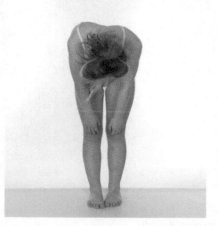

Figure 39.2   Clinical photograph showing the Adam's forward bend test.

Q: How would you describe the plain radiograph, and what is the most likely diagnosis?
This standing plain radiograph of the whole spine demonstrates a right thoracic curve with its apex at T7/8, with a Cobb angle measuring 56 degrees (Figure 39.3). Iliac crests demonstrate her to be Risser 2 (Table 39.1).

The most likely diagnosis is adolescent idiopathic scoliosis (AIS), a 3-dimensional spinal deformity with lateral curvature >10 degrees. It is defined as idiopathic scoliosis in children between 10 and 18 years of age and is the most common cause of scoliosis. 1–3% of children aged 10–16 have some degree of spinal curvature, but most do not require surgery. Fewer than 25% have pain at presentation. AIS is diagnosed when other causes of scoliosis, such as vertebral malformations, neuromuscular disorders and other syndromes have been excluded.

There is a 10:1 F:M preponderance of incidence of curves above 30 degrees.

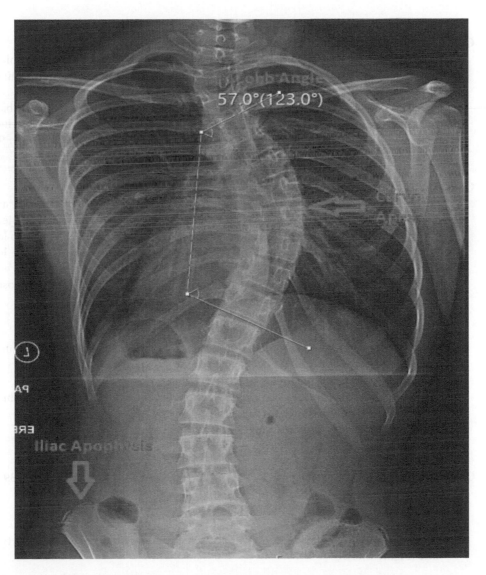

Figure 39.3   Plain radiograph whole spine showing right-sided scoliosis (labelled).

Table 39.1 Risser Grading

Risser Grade	Skeletal Findings and Maturity
0	No sign of calcification—correlates with skeletal immaturity
1	Initial appearance of ossification of the iliac apophysis calcified 0–25%—correlates with prepuberty and maximal rate of spinal growth
2	Ossification 25–50% across superior ilium—correlates with continued spinal growth
3	Ossification 50–75%—correlates with slowing of spinal growth
4	Ossification 75–100% without full fusion—correlates with near-complete spinal growth
5	Ossification fused to iliac crest relates to full maturity

Q: What is the pathophysiology of AIS?

The pathophysiology of AIS is unknown but suggested associations include mechanical, metabolic, hormonal, neuromuscular, growth and genetic abnormalities. AIS is a multi-factorial disease with genetic predisposing factors.

Back pain may be the presenting complaint. The association between scoliosis and back pain has been demonstrated in a retrospective study of 2442 patients with AIS, which found that 23% of patients with AIS had back pain at initial presentation, and another 9% developed back pain during the study.

Q: Which features would be indications for further imaging?

A key feature in the assessment of scoliosis is whether a curve is flexible or inflexible and whether a curve is structural or compensatory. If surgery is planned, AP bending views should be performed to see if smaller curves reduce. Curves which straighten out to less than 25 degrees on bending views are likely to be non-structural curves. They are less pronounced and develop later than the major curve.

MRI is indicated to rule out intraspinal abnormalities and should extend from posterior fossa to conus medullaris (normally around L1/2).

Indications for MRI include

- atypical curve patterns (left thoracic curve, apical kyphosis, short, dystrophic curve pattern),
- rapid progression on serial radiographs,
- structural abnormalities seen on plain radiograph (e.g. hemivertebra/block vertebra),
- neurological symptoms or severe pain,
- foot deformities (e.g. cavovarus) and
- asymmetrical abdominal reflexes

Q: What are the key features on a plain radiograph of a patient with scoliosis? (Figure 39.4)

Stable vertebrae

- The most proximal vertebrae that is most closely bisected by the central sacral vertical line (Figure 39.4).

Neutral vertebrae

- Rotationally neutral vertebrae (spinous process equal distance to pedicles on PA X-ray).

End vertebrae

- End vertebra is defined as the vertebra that is most tilted from the horizontal apical vertebra.

Apical vertebrae

- The apical vertebra is the disc/vertebra deviated farthest from the centre of the vertebral column.

Remember: The Cobb angle is measured between the 2 end vertebrae. Less than 10 degrees is defined as scoliosis. There is an interobserver error of 3–5 degrees.

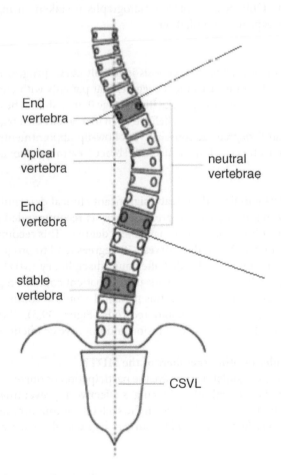

Figure 39.4   Coronal plane spinal parameters.

Q: Which features predict the progression of this condition, and what is its natural history?

A prospective study on the natural history of scoliosis reported that before skeletal maturity, curves >25 degrees continue to progress and should be monitored. After skeletal maturity, thoracic curves >50 degrees progress by 1–2 degrees/year and lumbar curves > 40 degrees progress by 1–2 degrees/year.

Rate of progression is related to skeletal maturity, as measured by Risser grading (Table 39.1). Risser 0–1 covers the first 2/3rd of pubertal growth and the greatest velocity of skeletal linear growth.

Progressive scoliosis can lead to worsening deformity, cosmesis and in severe cases, cardiorespiratory compromise. Around 10% of adolescents with idiopathic scoliosis will progress to a level requiring consideration of surgery.

Q: What should be the definitive management of patients with this condition?

Observation for AIS is the most common approach used for patients with mild deformity (Cobb angle <25 degrees). Depending on the degree of skeletal maturity, patients are assessed every 4 to 6 months to look for curve progression. The interval of follow-up will be determined on an individual basis, based on the age of the patient, degree of curve and skeletal maturity. Only posteroanterior radiographs are taken during each follow-up visit to minimise the exposure to radiation.

Bracing

The primary goal of bracing for scoliosis is to halt curve progression. The most widely accepted practice for brace treatment suggests that patients with curves of 25–45 degrees and in the most rapidly growing stage (Risser stage 0 or 1) should be offered a brace on initial evaluation. Curve progression is defined as an increase in the magnitude of the deformity by more than 5 degrees at consecutive follow-up appointments of between 4 and 6 months. Various factors can hinder successful brace treatment. Poor adherence is common.

Surgery

Surgery is generally indicated to treat a significant clinical deformity or to correct a scoliotic deformity that is likely to progress. Surgery is recommended in adolescents with a curve that has a Cobb angle greater than 45–50 degrees. This recommendation is derived from studies that have shown that curves >50 degrees tend to progress slowly after maturity. Management should be decided after multidisciplinary (MDT) discussion. Surgery should be preceded by appropriate work-up and patient counselling.

Given the degree of deformity in this patient, I would recommend a posterior spinal fusion using pedicle screws and contoured rods (Figure 39.5). The aim of surgery is to correct the deformity, achieve a solid fusion and improve cosmetic appearance.

Q: What are the roles of other members of the MDT?

Current best practice guidelines involve the participation of nurses, surgeons, physiotherapists, psychiatrists and orthotists. Bracing is effective at preventing progression into the surgical range (defined as ≥50 degrees) in the skeletally immature child (Risser 0, 1, 2) and can lead to a 50% reduction in need for surgery by skeletal maturity.

Exam Tips

- This is a core topic that could come up in the long cases, and so you should know it in depth. There are classification systems of AIS (Lenke and King-Moe), but in-depth knowledge of these is beyond what is needed for the FRCS exam. See the references for more insight into the surgical management of AIS.

- The Adams forward bend test assesses the degree of rotational deformity associated with the scoliosis. The patient is asked to bend forward at the waist with the knees straight and the palms together. Look down the back for the presence of asymmetry in the rib cage (rib prominence) or deformities along the back indicative of a structural scoliosis. A non-structural curve (postural scoliosis) normally disappears on bending forwards.
- Always remember to inspect gait and to look around for walking aids and things such as shoe lifts. These are easy marks and frequently missed.
- Don't forget to mention the MDT!

SUGGESTED READINGS

1. Altaf F, Gibson A, Dannawi Z, et al. Adolescent idiopathic scoliosis. BMJ. 2013;346:f2508.
2. Weinstein SL, Dolan LA, Cheng JC, et al. Adolescent idiopathic scoliosis. Lancet. 2008;371:1527–37.
3. Lenke L, Edwards C, Bridwell K. The Lenke classification of adolescent idiopathic scoliosis: how it organizes curve patterns as a template to perform selective fusions of the spine. Spine (Phila Pa 1976). 2003;28(20):S199–207.

40

NEUROMUSCULAR SCOLIOSIS

Q: An 8-year-old boy presents to your clinic with a known diagnosis of cerebral palsy (CP), GMFCS 3. He has a scoliosis which has been monitored for the last 5 years. Initial treatment was with bracing. The child's parents now report that the child is experiencing back pain and has difficulty balancing when sitting. The sitting X-ray (XR) is shown. Please comment.

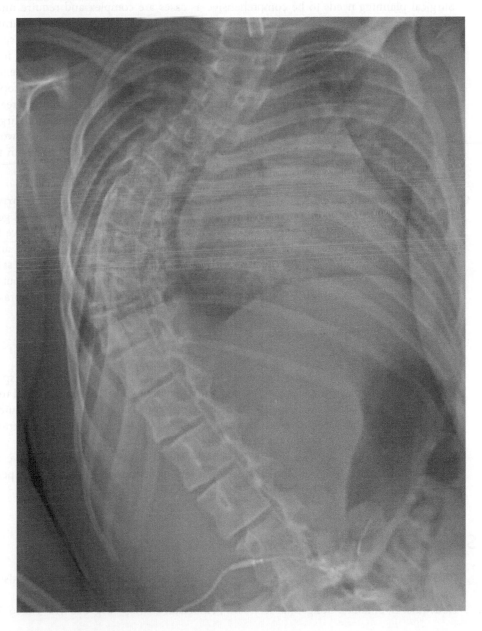

DOI: 10.1201/9781003201304-47

This is an AP XR demonstrating a long c-shaped scoliosis. I would like to elicit more from the history in terms of the functional status of the child and how this may have changed since the last review. I would like to examine the child, paying particular attention to the overall strength and mobility of the child, as well as more specifically paying attention to the spine in terms of curve flexibility, overall balance and any pelvic obliquity. I would like to measure the cobb angle of the curve on the current radiograph and compare it to previous films to assess curve progression.

Q: The curve measures 80 degrees and has progressed 10 degrees since the last review 1 year ago. The family would like to consider surgery. What issues would you discuss with them prior to decision making?

Surgical planning needs to be comprehensive as cases are complex and require multi-disciplinary input. The multisystem pathology of CP patients requires careful optimisation. Particular attention needs to be paid to respiratory function, as performing a spinal fusion in a skeletally immature patient may impair growth of the thorax and lung function. Pre-existing neurological disorders such as epilepsy may be exacerbated by general anaesthetic (GA). Disorders of the gastrointestinal (GI) system such as gastro-oesophageal reflux disease are common in CP patients and place the child at significantly increased risk of aspiration and poor oral intake with resultant malnutrition. The risks of surgery including catastrophic neurological injury and medical/anaesthetic complications would also need to be outlined in detail. Post-operative complications are also higher in this patient population.

Q: What are the main surgical goals, and what surgical procedure would you perform?

In curves larger than 50 degrees in CP, surgery should be considered. The overall goals of surgery are to achieve a balanced spine, prevent further deterioration of the curve and improve quality of life. A careful assessment of pelvic obliquity would be necessary, and I would like to perform a whole-spine MRI and CT under GA pre-operatively to assess the bony anatomy, pedicles, termination of the conus and position of the cord throughout the length of the spine. Ultimately, I would consider a long posterior fusion from thorax to pelvis to control the curve and the pelvic obliquity.

Exam Tips

- Neuromuscular scoliosis may be caused by a number of disorders of the brain, spinal cord and muscular system (e.g. CP, spinal muscular atrophy). These curves tend to be long c-shaped curves, are associated with pelvic obliquity and progress more quickly than adolescent idiopathic curves. They are at higher risk of operative and perioperative complications.
- Surgical goals are on a case-by-case basis depending on the severity of the curve and functional status. Surgery tends to involve a long thoracolumbar construct ± pelvic fixation depending on the functional status and needs of the patient.

SUGGESTED READINGS

1. Cloake T, Gardner A. The management of scoliosis in children with cerebral palsy: a review. J Spine Surg. 2016;2(4):299–309.
2. Hedequist D, Emans J. Congenital scoliosis. J Am Acad Orthop Surg. 2004;12(4):266–75.

41

PAEDIATRIC SPONDYLOLISTHESIS

Q: A 14-year-old netball player comes with her mother to your clinic complaining of worsening lower back pain. Her axial CT taken at the L5 level is shown. **Can you comment?**

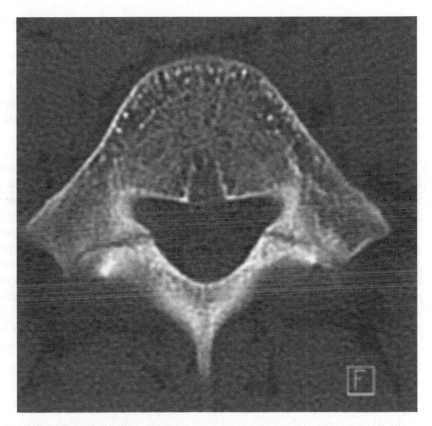

The CT shows an axial slice of the patient's L5 vertebra. There appear to be bilateral lytic defects across the pars interarticualris. Given the patient's history of worsening back and leg pain, I would be concerned about a pars defect. I would like to see a standing 36-inch X-ray (XR) to assess for any spondylolisthesis and to obtain an MRI scan given the history of leg pain to assess compression of the nerve roots.

Q: Can you tell me about the natural history of this condition in the paediatric population?

Pars defects represent a spectrum of disease and have different aetiologies. The pars itself may be sclerotic because of a stress reaction. Further progression may lead to a fracture defined as spondylolysis. This may then cause the vertebrae to translate with respect to the vertebra below, defined as spondylolisthesis. This is most common in the paediatric population at the L5/S1 level. Translation of the vertebra may put the L5 nerve root at risk, causing radicular symptoms as described by this patient.

DOI: 10.1201/9781003201304-48

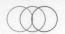

Q: Are you aware of any classification systems associated with this condition?
The Wiltse–Newman Classification describes type I dysplastic, type II Isthmic, type III degenerative, type IV traumatic and type V neoplastic. Dysplastic pars defects are secondary to congenital abnormalities, for example hypoplastic facets. Isthmic spondylolisthesis can be due to fatigue fracture, elongation due to healed stress fractures and acute fractures, most likely the cause in this individual. The Meyerding classification describes the grade of spondylolisthesis based on the percentage slippage of one vertebral body with respect to the other. In 2006, Mac-Thiong and Labelle proposed a surgical classification system based on slip severity, dysplasia and sagittal alignment.

Q: The upright XR demonstrates no obvious spondylolisthesis. How would you manage this patient?
Most symptomatic patients with this condition can be managed successfully non-operatively. The CT scan demonstrates bilateral lysis of the pars, and the patient is therefore at risk of developing spondylolisthesis. Nonetheless, given the lack of dynamic instability evident on the XR, a period—about 3 months—of activity restriction and physiotherapy would be reasonable. If this fails to improve the symptoms, then bracing in a thoraco lumbar sacral orthosis brace may be tried.

Q: The patient returns to your clinic after 6 months of non-operative management complaining that the pain is worse, and she has developed right-sided pain radiating to the lateral aspect of her leg and dorsum of the foot. Upright XR demonstrates a Meyerding Grade I spondylolisthesis. How would you proceed with management?
Although studies have suggested a benign course in low-grade spondylolisthesis, this patient has progressive pain symptoms and onset of neurology. Surgical options include bilateral pars repair with screws or tension band wiring. Alternatively, posterior instrumented fusion and decompression would successfully stabilise the slip and decompress the nerve root. Studies have demonstrated that in patients who fail non-operative management, surgical fusion results in a high success rate. Evidence is suggestive that high-grade spondylolisthesis may be treated with circumferential fusion, that is anterior fusion with an interbody device and posterior fusion in preference to posterior-only approaches.

Exam Tips

- Although candidates are not routinely asked to quote classification systems, knowledge of the above systems to classify spondylolisthesis would help to gain higher marks in the exam. The surgical classification system by Mac-Thiong and Labelle mentioned earlier incorporates sagittal spino-pelvic balance and attempts to offer a guide to surgical treatment.
- The majority of paediatric patients presenting with this condtion can be managed non-operatively. Nonetheless, recognition of the onset of neurological symptoms as an indication to operate is key.

SUGGESTED READINGS

1. Crawford CH, Larson AN, Gates M, et al. Current evidence regarding the treatment of paediatric lumbar spondylolisthesis: a report from the Scoliosis Research Society Evidence Based Medicine Committee. Spine Deform. 2017;5(5):284–302.
2. Mac-Thiong J-M, Labelle H. A proposal for a surgical classification of paediatric lumbo-sacral spondylolisthesis based on current literature. Eur Spine J. 2006;15(10):1425–35.

42

CONGENITAL SCOLIOSIS

You are in the paediatric spinal clinic. You are asked to see a 9-year-old boy, whose mother has noticed a gradual curvature of his spine over the previous 2 years. He is in mainstream schooling, but his mother reports that he was slightly delayed in achieving his developmental educational milestones. He is also reported to be 'quite clumsy', with a history of recurrent trips and falls.

His past medical history includes a hypospadias. Your neurological examination is grossly normal. You request a 3-foot standing view of the whole spine (Figure 42.1).

Q: What is the diagnosis?

This patient has an apex left-sided congenital thoracolumbar scoliosis secondary to a hemivertebra in the lower thoracic spine.

Congenital scoliosis is a failure of vertebral formation, segmentation or a combination of the two, arising from abnormal vertebral development during weeks 4 to 6 of gestation. The associated spinal deformity can be of varying severity and can result in a stable or progressive deformity based on the type and location of the abnormal vertebra.

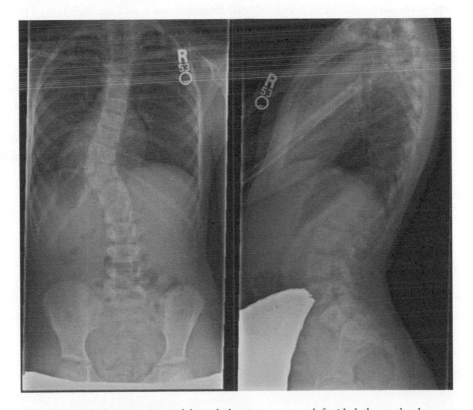

Figure 42.1 X-ray whole-spine PA and lateral showing an apex left-sided thoracolumbar congenital scoliosis with associated hemivertebra.

DOI: 10.1201/9781003201304-49

Q: What other physical examination should be performed?

Congenital scoliosis can be associated with a number of underlying conditions, in isolation or in association with the VACTERL (vertebral anomalies, anorectal atresia, cardiac anomalies, tracheoesophageal fistula and/or [o]esophageal atresia, renal and limb anomalies) syndrome. Therefore, a thorough cardiopulmonary examination should be performed.

The musculoskeletal system should be examined closely for other anomalies in the cervical spine (e.g. Klippel-Feil syndrome), upper extremity (e.g. Sprengel's deformity or radial deficiency) and/or lower extremity (e.g. developmental dysplasia of the hip).

Genitourinary abnormalities are observed in 20–40% of these children. External genitalia should be examined after appropriate explanation to the patient or carer in the presence of a suitable clinical chaperone.

Q: How can congenital scoliosis be classified, and what is the clinical relevance of this classification?

Congenital scoliosis is classically described as a failure of segmentation, formation or a mixed form (Figure 42.2). Approximately 80% of anomalies may be classified as either failures of segmentation or formation, with 20% being a mixed form.

Segmentation defects involve bony bars between adjacent segments. A block vertebra results from bilateral segmentation defects with the fusion of the disc spaces between the involved vertebrae. A unilateral bar typically occurs on the concave side of a curve. A unilateral unsegmented bar is a bony bar fusing both the disc spaces and/or facets on 1 side of the spine.

The unsegmented bar does not contain growth plates and therefore does not grow. Failure of formation produces either a wedge vertebra or a hemivertebra. A wedge vertebra represents partial failure of vertebral body formation on 1 side but maintains 2 pedicles. In contrast, a hemivertebra represents a complete failure of formation of half the vertebra. There are 3 main types of hemivertebrae: fully segmented (65%), partially segmented (22%) and non-segmented/ incarcerated (12%).

A fully segmented hemivertebra possesses a normal disc both above and below the anomaly. A partially segmented hemivertebra is fused to the neighbouring vertebra on 1 side with an open disc space on the opposite side. An incarcerated hemivertebra has no intervening disc space between the adjacent vertebrae.

The determinants of curve progression depend on the type of abnormality, its location and the age of the patient. The anomaly that is at the most at risk for progression is the unilateral

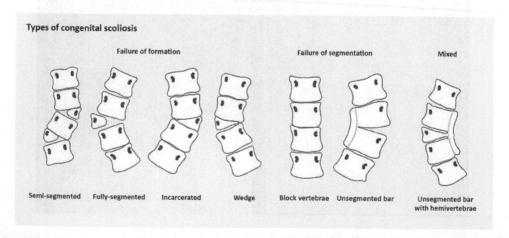

Figure 42.2 Classification of congenital scoliosis.

bar with contralateral hemivertebra, followed by a unilateral bar, a hemivertebra, a wedge vertebra and a block vertebra, which is the least likely to cause any significant deformity.

Q: What other imaging should be requested?

CT scan of the whole spine can be useful in the identification of bony anatomy and for surgical planning but should be used sparingly due to the long-term risks of radiation exposure. MRI scan of the whole spine should be requested in all patients with a suspected congenital scoliosis to identify possible neural axis abnormality (found in 20–40%). These include Chiari malformation, tethered cord, diastematomyelia and syringomyelia (MRI may require formal sedation in infants or prolonged coaxing/persuasion in older children!).

Renal ultrasound/MRI and echocardiogram should be performed to exclude other systemic abnormalities.

Q: How should these patients be treated?

These patients should be treated in a multidisciplinary fashion, with the involvement of physicians, paediatricians and physiotherapists.

Observation is appropriate for patients with an absence of radiographic progression or clinical symptoms (more likely with incarcerated hemivertebrae or non-segmental hemivertebrae) These curves are usually inflexible and unresponsive to bracing.

Surgical correction is indicated for deformities that are increasing in severity or an anomaly with a high risk for progression. This is classically via posterior instrumented fusion, although anterior approaches can also be used in some cases. All types of fusion before skeletal maturity impact growth potential to an extent. Growth rods (such as the MAGnetic Expansion Control [Magec] system) may be used to control deformity during spinal growth and to delay arthrodesis (fusion) to maximise growth potential.

Q: What are the risks of surgical management?

These include risks of neurological injury due to over distraction/over correction, as well as risks of paralysis due to screw misplacement. Other specific complications after scoliosis surgery include the 'crankshaft phenomenon' (a progressive rotational and angular spinal deformity that can occur after isolated posterior spinal surgery) and superior mesenteric artery (SMA) syndrome (a rare proximal bowel obstruction due to the contraction of the angle between the SMA and the aorta during scoliosis surgery).

Exam Tips

- Most AIS curves are right-sided. Any left-sided curve (such as in this vignette) should instantly make you think about underlying pathology and warrant an MRI scan of the whole spine.
- The details of the surgical management of congenital scoliosis are complex and beyond the scope of the FRCS examination. You should be aware of the classification of congenital scoliosis and of the management options in general terms.

SUGGESTED READINGS

1. Williams BA, Matsumoto H, McCalla DJ, et al. Development and initial validation of the Classification of Early-Onset Scoliosis (CEOS). J Bone Joint Surg Am. 2014;96:1359–67.
2. Pahys J, Guille J. What's new in congenital scoliosis? J Pediatr Orthop. 2018;38(3):e172–9.

SECTION 8
INFECTION

43

EPIDURAL ABSCESS

Q: A 45-year-old female presents to the ED with a 6-month history of progressively worsening low back pain. In the last 2 weeks she has experienced a worsening pain radiating to her right leg and upper back. She undergoes a CT scan, which is shown. Please comment.

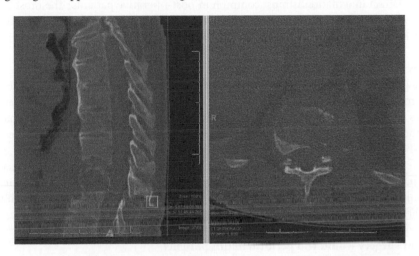

This is a sagittal and axial CT slice of the thoracic spine. This demonstrates gross destruction of at least one of the lower thoracic vertebral bodies. There appears to be focal kyphosis. I am concerned about infection and tumour. I would like to elicit more from the history including risk factors for both, perform a full neurological examination and obtain and MRI scan with gadolinium contrast.

Q: The patient has a history of intravenous drug use (IVDU) and diabetes. Examination reveals she is haemodynamically stable but has a high white cell count. Blood cultures are positive for *Staphylococcus aureus* . She is in too much pain to mobilise but has grade 4/5 power throughout all myotomes in her lower limbs. MRI scan is as shown. Please comment on the MRI.

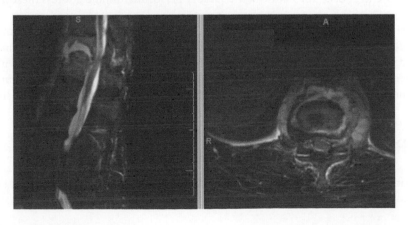

DOI: 10.1201/9781003201304-51

The MRI demonstrates what appears to be a paravertebral collection. The axial imaging does not demonstrate any obvious cord compression, but further axial cuts would need to be reviewed to exclude this.

Q: What is the pathogenesis of this patient's pathology?

This patient is suffering from vertebral osteomyelitis. Intravenous drug abuse and diabetes are amongst the most common risk factors for this condition. In cases of native vertebral osteomyelitis, infection tends to occur most commonly at the vertebral endplates via haematogenous seeding. Spread is from the endplate to the disc and then to the opposite endplate. Direct inoculation is most common in post-operative patients. The most common pathogen is staphylococcus aureus, followed by *Staphylococcus epidermidis*. In the IVDU patient population, *Pseudomonas* is also common.

Q: How would you manage this patient?

This patient has a significant infection in their lower thoracic vertebral bodies. From the neurological assessment, it is unclear as to whether the patient has any myelopathic features but appears to have well-preserved power. The patient needs surgical management as the spine is unstable given the extensive destruction of the vertebral bodies. Based on the imaging shown, there does not appear to be any obvious compressive epidural abscess. The patient requires reviewing by the infectious diseases team and anaesthetic team. Assuming the patient is clinically well and has not been started on antibiotics, these should be withheld until intraoperative sampling can be taken in order to achieve the highest yield.

Q: What surgery would you perform in this patient?

Given the degree of vertebral destruction present here, along with the lower thoracic/ junctional location of this infection, this case would most likely require anterior support in the form of an interbody device, augmented by a posterior construct also. If further scrutiny of the MRI showed any sign of epidural abscess formation, I would also perform a posterior decompression.

Exam Tips

- The indications for surgical management in vertebral osteomyelitis are neurological compromise and instability. Neurological compromise may occur because of compression of the neural elements either from an epidural abscess or instability causing collapse/kyphosis. The nature of the surgery performed should address these issues as key goals.
- Post-operative infection may be superficial incisional or deep incisional (involving fascial or muscle layers) or involve an organ space (Public Health England guidelines) and should always cause concern when faced with this presentation. Patients with post-operative vertebral osteomyelitis have been shown to represent a different patient cohort to native vertebral osteomyelitis and have better patient outcomes and disease severity.

REFERENCE

1. Breuninger M, Yagdiran A, Willinger A, et al. Vertebral osteomyelitis after spine surgery: a disease with distinct characteristics. Spine. 2020;45(20):1426–34.

44

SPINAL TUBERCULOSIS

A 28-year-old female presents to the emergency department with a 1-week history of central posterior neck pain, cough and intermittent fevers. She is a married office worker of South-East Asian origin and had immigrated to the UK 3 years previously from India. On arrival in the UK, she reported a negative tuberculosis (TB) polymerase chain reaction result. Her medical history is positive for diabetes mellitus type 2.

Bloods were drawn on admission (as follows): WCC. 9.0 x 10⁹/L, CRP: 18 mg/L, erythrocyte sedimentation rate 16 mm/hr.

Bedside observations were as follows: heat rate (HR): 86 bpm, RR: 18 b/minute, T: 37.8°

On examination, her neurological findings are normal. An X-ray of her chest is requested (Figure 44.1).

A PA chest radiograph was performed. This was reported as showing a right paratracheal lesion (labelled) with multiple small pulmonary nodules.

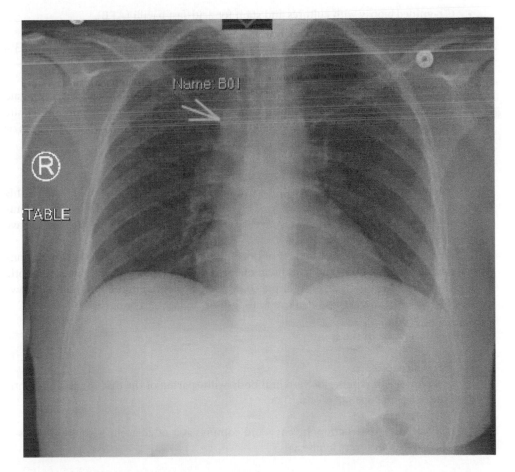

Figure 44.1 X-ray chest showing right paratracheal lesion with multiple small pulmonary nodules.

DOI: 10.1201/9781003201304-52

Q: What is the likely diagnosis, and what further investigations would you request?

The most likely diagnosis is of TB infection with possible spinal involvement. Blood cultures should be taken to exclude other bacterial and/or fungal infective organisms.

Patients at risk of TB include those at the extremes of age, diabetics, smokers, cancer patients and alcoholics. The primary route of infection is pulmonary or genitourinary, and 50% of all TB patients have a primary lung foci or history of pulmonary tuberculosis.

Of those with active disease, approximately 10% are impacted by skeletal tuberculosis, while 5% of all TB patients have spinal involvement.

It is important to assess the extent of vertebral involvement. This can be achieved with plain radiographs and CT scans of the cervical spine. MRI scan with gadolinium contrast of the cervical and thoracic spine can identify fluid collection and neural element compression.

Bone scan may show other skeletal sites of involvement; however, there is limited evidence that it can accurately differentiate between infection and metastasis. Positron emission tomography (PET) may have a role in identifying hypermetabolic abscesses to target for a higher yield to obtain tissue biopsy specimens.

Diagnosis

- CT-guided biopsy with cultures and stain for acid-fast bacilli (AFB).
  - Mycobacteria (AFB) may take 10 weeks to grow in culture.
  - Polymerase chain reaction allows for faster identification (95% sensitivity and 93% accuracy).

Tissue diagnosis is the gold standard diagnostic test for spinal tuberculosis. All tissue samples should be sent for culture, histopathology and polymerase chain reaction. Tissue can be obtained via CT-guided needle biopsy or surgical biopsy if image guidance fails or surgical management is imminent.

Q: What are the classical imaging findings in spinal TB?

Of patients with active TB, 66% will have an abnormal CXR (Figure 44.1), and so this should be ordered in any patient where TB is a possibility, especially those with immunocompromise, and those who have travelled to or been in contact with those who have travelled to endemic regions.

Spinal TB has a characteristic loss of bone density in the anterior spine. Lytic lesions involve the vertebral body and paradiscal margins. Radiographs can also reveal kyphotic deformities through a single or multiple contiguous or non-contiguous vertebrae. However, X-rays often reveal these classical findings only in later stages of the disease.

Plain radiographs of the spine

- Early infection
  - Involvement of anterior vertebral body with sparing of the disc space (differentiates from pyogenic infection)
- Late infection
  - Disk space destruction, lucency and compression of adjacent vertebral bodies—can result in severe kyphosis.

CT (Figure 44.2)

- Findings
  - Types of destruction can be divided into
    - Fragmentary, osteolytic (most common), subperiosteal, sclerotic

MRI with gadolinium contrast (Figure 44.3)—low signal on T1-weighted images, bright signal on T2-weighted images.

Her CT scan (Figure 44.2) showed osteolytic fracture of the C2 vertebra with translation of at the fracture site. MRI scan showed C2 vertebral fracture with surrounding oedema without significant cervical stenosis.

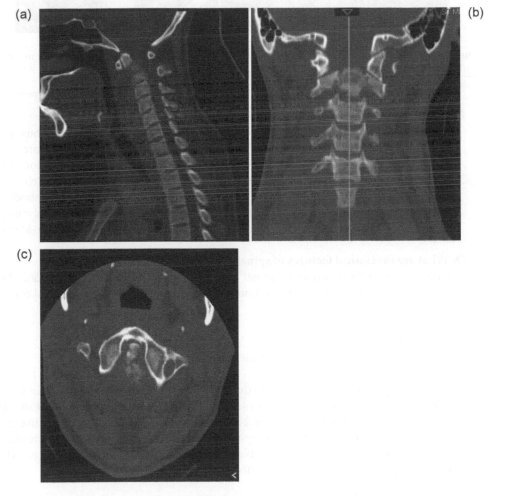

Figure 44.2 CT scan cervical spine—(a) sagittal, (b) coronal and (c) axial (C2)—showing osteolytic fracture of the C2 vertebra with translation at the fracture site.

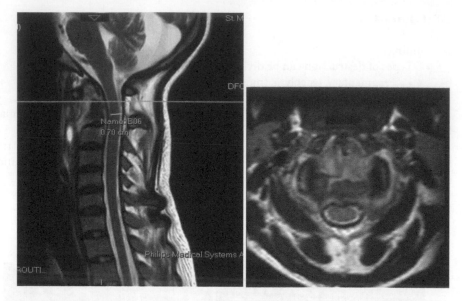

Figure 44.3   MRI scan (T2-weighted) showing C2 vertebral fracture with surrounding oedema without significant cervical stenosis.

Q: What is the pattern of spinal involvement in TB?

Spinal TB is a secondary infection, which generally occurs via haematogenous spread. Unlike most infections of the spine, 95% of spinal tuberculosis begins in the anterior vertebral body. The infection spreads from either arterial spread in paradiscal region or from the valveless venous plexus (Batson's paravertebral plexus) into the central vertebral body.

The infection spreads under the ALL and into the posterior vertebral body. The intervertebral disc is often last to be affected. If left untreated, the bony involvement in spinal tuberculosis eventually destroys the anterior vertebral bodies, leading to kyphosis.

Q: What are the clinical features of spinal TB?

Only 20–30% of the patients with spinal TB have constitutional symptoms (chronic illness, malaise, night sweats). It has an insidious progression with three major clinical features:

1. Cold abscesses
2. Neurologic deficit
3. Long-term kyphotic deformity of the spine

Neurologic deficit occurs in approximately 10–20% of individuals. This manifestation is more common in cervical and thoracic disease caused by the proximity of the spinal cord and is rarer in the lumbar spine. Neurologic symptoms can progress to myelopathy and paraplegia or even tetraplegia if cephalad enough. The cord itself can become infected, and cord oedema can also be responsible for neurologic deficits. In rare instances, arteritis of the spinal artery can result in thrombosis and ischemia of the spinal cord.

Q: How would you definitively manage this patient?

Medical management is the mainstay of management of spinal TB in absence of radiological features of instability or neurological deficit. Pharmacologic agents include rifampicin (R), isoniazid (I), pyrazanamide (P) and ethambutol (E).

Spinal orthosis (bracing) can be used in addition to medical management for pain control and prevention of deformity. However, this has more utility in the thoracic spine (rather than the cervical spine) due to the inherent stability given by the rib cage and sternum.

A 2006 Cochrane review did not find sufficient evidence to conclusively recommend routine surgical treatment for the treatment of spinal tuberculosis. Current indications for surgical management include worsening neurological deficit, acute severe paraplegia and pan-vertebral involvement and risk of progressive instability with/without subluxation/dislocation (± neurological deficit).

The surgical approach depends on the location of the infection, the presence of deformity as well as the presence of neurological symptoms and spinal cord compression.

The major options can be divided into

- **anterior decompression/corpectomy ± posterior instrumented stabilisation and**
- **posterior only instrumented stabilisation ± decompression.**

Posterior kyphosis correction can be performed via bony osteotomies to correct late-stage kyphosis, particularly in the lumbar spine. (See spinal osteotomy q. 30.)

5. What are the possible complications of surgery?

- Deformity (kyphosis)
  - This is most commonly associated with anterior decompression and grafting alone.
  - The lowest risk of progressive deformity is after both anterior and posterior fusion (can be single stage or two stage).
- Retropharyngeal abscess affects swallowing/hoarseness
- TB arteritis and pseudoaneurysm
- Sinus formation
- **Pott's paraplegia**
  - Spinal cord injury (SCI) can be caused by abscess/bony sequestra or meningomyelitis
  - Abscess/bony sequestra has a better prognosis than meningomyelitis as the cause of SCI

Exam Tips

- Remember that early infection in TB shows the involvement of anterior vertebral body with sparing of the disc space (this is a key finding can differentiate from pyogenic infection).
- TB should be high on your list of differential diagnoses when faced with this history and you should consider it as a possible diagnosis in any patient with possible signs of infection. An in-depth knowledge of the surgical management of TB of the spine is not required (unless you are in gold-medal territory).
- Remember the useful acronym for the medical management of TB—**R.I.P.E** (see the earlier dicussion).
- You should be able to spot the pathognomonic signs on radiograph and MRI scan. These patients should always be managed in an MDT fashion along with the medical team. Marks will be given for thorough knowledge of how to examine these patients' neurological status thoroughly. If a patient seems to have a stable pattern on CT/MRI scan and has no neurological abnormality, make sure to mention that you would get

sequential imaging to make sure they don't get progressive instability which would necessitate surgical management.

SUGGESTED READINGS

1. Jutte PC, van Loenhout-Rooyackers JH. Routine surgery in addition to chemotherapy for treating spinal tuberculosis. Cochrane Database Syst Rev. 2006;(5):CD004532.
2. Khanna K, Sabharwal S. Spinal tuberculosis: a comprehensive review for the modern spine surgeon. Spine J. 2019;19(11):1858–70.
3. Rajasekaran S, Chand D, Soundararajan R, et al. Spinal tuberculosis: current concepts. Global Spine J. 2018;8(4S):96S–108S.
4. Panditaa A, Madhuripanb N, Panditac S, et al. Challenges and controversies in the treatment of spinal tuberculosis. Clin Tuberc Other Mycobact Dis. 2020;19:100151.

SECTION 9
OTHER USEFUL CASES

45

ATLANTOAXIAL SUBLUXATION IN RHEUMATOID ARTHRITIS

Q: A 40-year-old female presents to your clinic complaining of worsening neck pain. She describes intermittent loss of balance and reduced manual dexterity. Her past medical history includes rheumatoid arthritis (RA). **How do you proceed?**

I am concerned that the patient's rheumatoid disease is affecting her cervical spine. I would like to examine her clinically, looking specifically for features of myelopathy, and obtain upright flexion-extension radiographs.

Flexion extension radiographs are shown. Please comment.

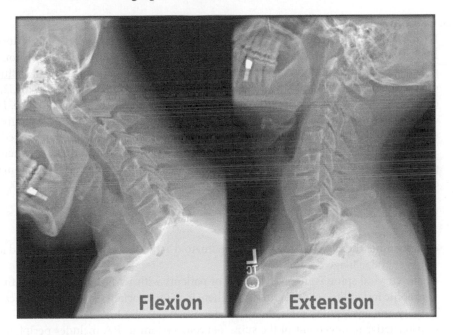

Flexion   Extension

There appears to be a degree of instability between the atlas and the dens between the flexion and extension views. This is suggestive of atlantoaxial subluxation, the most common rheumatoid c-spine problem, present in about 70% of patients. This can exist as anterior subluxation (0%), posterior subluxation (7%) or lateral subluxation (10%). I would assess this by measuring the ADI and posterior atlanto-dens interval (PADI), the latter of which equates to space available for the cord. In anterior subluxation if the ADI is greater than 3mm, this is abnormal. If the PADI is less than 15mm, this is also concerning. If the PADI is less than 13mm, this is an indication for surgery due to the risk of cord compression. Posterior atlanto-axial subluxation occurs if the arch of C1 is incompetent or the dens is eroded.

There are two other major patterns of cervical instability. Basilar invagination, or cranial settling, describes the migration of the dens through the foramen magnum secondary to C1 lateral mass erosion. Subaxial subluxation is due to synovitis of the uncovertebral

DOI: 10.1201/9781003201304-54

joint and facet instability due to bone and soft tissue erosion. This is concerning if subluxation is present >3mm or if there are multiple subluxations present.

Q: On the upright X-ray (XR), the ADI measures 4mm and the PADI 12mm. How would you manage this patient?

This patient describes symptoms of myelopathy and has cervical parameters which are concerning for cord compression. I would like to obtain a CT to assess bony changes and an MRI scan to evaluate pannus formation. The indications for surgical intervention in the rheumatoid neck are intractable pain, neurologic dysfunction, subaxial subluxation and atlanto-axial subluxation greater than 8mm. If the preceding investigations and examination were suggestive of cord compression/myelopathy, I would offer the patient surgery. Patients with neurological deficit should be offered surgery given the high mortality with non-operative management.

Q: What surgery would you offer?

I would offer a posterior C1/C2 fusion.

Q: Can you describe the management of basilar invagination?

Basilar invagination can be measured radiographically using several criteria including McRae's line and the Ranawat line (see the following figure and table). Once confirmed radiologically as present, progressive radiological parameters or neurological dysfunction are an indication for surgery. I would offer a posterior fusion of the occiput to C2. However, first, I would need to assess if the invagination was reducible or irreducible. I would do this intraoperatively by placing the patient in traction and adding 2.5 lb progressively under an image intensifier. Eighty per cent of cases of basilar invagination are reducible. After reduction, I would perform a posterior occiput to C2 fusion. If it was irreducible, the patient would require an occiput to C2 fusion with a laminectomy and foramen magnum decompression.

Exam Tips

- Remember the systemic features of rheumatoid arthritis as this question could lead on to general management of RA.
- The cervical spine is involved in 23% of patients with RA. Many patients with radiographic instability are asymptomatic. There is a 50% mortality at 1 year if cervical instability and myelopathy remain untreated.
- Alternative involvement of the spine/nervous system in RA includes peripheral neuropathy, carpal tunnel syndrome, vasculitis, vertebrobasilar insufficiency, spinal infections secondary to immunosuppression and osteoporotic fractures.

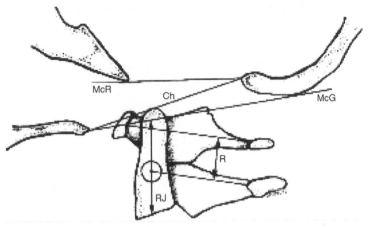

Cranial Settling Criteria

Line	Definition	Abnormal
McRae's line (McR)	Ant. to post. aspect of foramen magnum	Any protrusion of odontoid
Chamberlain's line (Ch)	From posterior aspect of hard palate to posterior lip of the foramen magnum	>3 mm of odontoid protrusion
McGregor line (McG)	Post. aspect of hard palate to inf. aspect of most caudal portion of occiput	>5 mm of odontoid protrusion
Ranawat Line (R)	Line 1 = from ant. to most posterior aspect of C1 Line 2 = vertical line from center of C2 pedicle (sclerotic ring) upward to intersect at right angles with previous line (line1)	R <13 mm abnormal Advantage: not dependent on visualising hard palate or dens which may be eroded
Wackenheim's clival canal line	Line which joins the dorsum sella to the tip of the clivus	Odontoid should be tangential or below this line
Redlund-Johnell (RJ)	OAA index of cranial settling = distance from McG to the sagittal midpoint at base of axis	<34 mm in men <29 mm in women

REFERENCE

1. Nguyen HV, Ludwig SC, Silber J, et al. Rheumatoid arthritis of the cervical spine. Spine J. 2004;4(3):329–34.

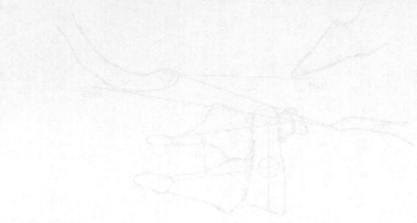

46

KLIPPEL-FEIL/SPRENGEL'S DEFORMITY

You are referred a 9-year-old girl from her GP. Her parents are concerned that she may have a scoliosis, although she herself denies any pain or functional impairment. She has full, pain-free range of movement in her upper limbs and no neurological impairment.

She has no other reported medical problems and has reached all her developmental milestones to this stage.

On inspection, she has a smaller scapula on the right side compared to the left (Figure 46.1) and a relatively short neck. She has a limited range of movement on cervical spine extension (when attempting to look towards the ceiling). Lateral X-rays of her cervical spine (Figure 46.2a) and PA X-ray of her whole spine (Figure 46.2b) are shown.

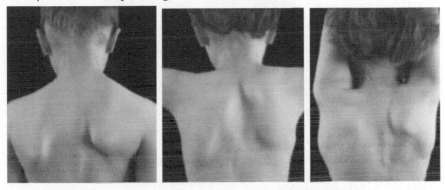

Figure 46.1 Clinical photograph showing asymmetry of scapula size.

(a)

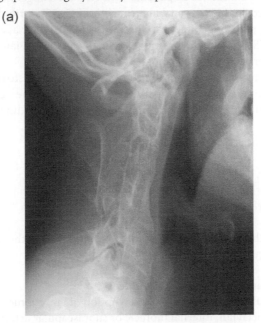

Figure 46.2a Lateral cervical X-ray showing fusion across all cervical vertebrae.

DOI: 10.1201/9781003201304-55

(b)

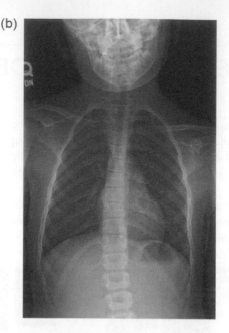

Figure 46.2b   AP X-ray whole-spine showing mild thoracolumbar scoliosis.

Q: What is the diagnosis?

The patient has a right-sided Sprengel's deformity (small and undescended scapula) and Klippel-Feil syndrome (KFS).

KFS is a congenital defect in the formation or segmentation of the cervical spine. The most associated anomalies in patients with KFS are congenital scoliosis (60% of cases), spina bifida occulta (45%), renal abnormalities (35–55%), rib deformity (20–30%), deafness (30–40%) and congenital heart disease (8–14%). Other associated conditions include high scapula (Sprengel deformity, present in 1/3 of cases), jaw anomalies, partial loss of hearing and torticollis.

It is characterised by the presence of congenital synostosis (fusion) of some or all cervical vertebrae. This congenital vertebral fusion of the cervical spine results from faulty segmentation along the embryo's developing axis during the first 3–8 weeks of gestation.

The diagnosis is based on a classical clinical triad:

* Short neck
* Low posterior hairline
* Limited neck movement

Patients with KFS are often asymptomatic; nevertheless, they may develop spontaneous neurologic sequelae as a result of their bony anomalies.

Q: What is the cause of Sprengel's shoulder?

Sprengel's shoulder is caused by an interruption of embryonic subclavian blood supply at the level of subclavian, internal thoracic or suprascapular artery.

Q: What further imaging would be required?
Plain radiographs of the cervical spine (AP, lateral, and odontoid views) are recommended. KFS can be associated with abnormalities of the atlantoaxial spine (C1–C2). The most common is basilar invagination (superior migration of the tip of the dens). The tip of the odontoid process is normally about 5mm below a point known as McCrea's line; basilar invagination is diagnosed when the tip crosses this line (Figure 46.3; see q. 45 (Atlantoaxial subuxation in Rheumatoid arthritis).

MRI of the whole spine should also be performed to exclude other spinal abnormalities with can accompany KFS.

Q: How can KFS be classified?
There are three subtypes as outlined by Feil et al. in the original description of the condition:

- Type I—single congenitally fused cervical segment
- type II—multiple non-contiguous, congenitally fused segments
- type III—multiple contiguous, congenitally fused cervical segments

Female patients are predominantly type I, while males are largely type III. Axial neck symptoms are highly associated with type I patients, whereas predominant radicular and myelopathic symptoms are associated with types II and III.

Q: What is the genetic background of this condition?
KFS may result from mutations or disruptions in genes regulating segmentation and re-segmentation. Although most cases of KFS are sporadic, there are at least 4 genetic forms of KFS with dominant or recessive inheritance. Most cases of KFS are thought to be due to a mutation in the SGM1 gene on Chromosome 8.

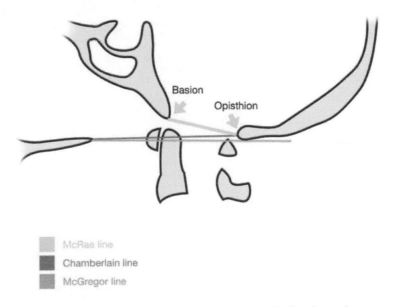

Figure 46.3 McRae line is a radiographic line drawn on a lateral skull radiograph or on a midsagittal section of CT or MRI that connects the anterior and posterior margins of the foramen magnum (basion to opisthion).

Q: How should this patient be managed?

This condition is often identified as an incidental finding when investigating possible scoliosis. Non-operative management with regular radiographic evaluation is the mainstay of treatment in most cases. Asymptomatic patients with fusions of 1–2 disc spaces below C3 can participate in contact sports while those with lesions affecting C2 should be advised to avoid contact sports.

Surgical decompression and posterior fusion should be reserved for those patients with basilar invagination, chronic pain, myelopathy, associated atlantoaxial instability or adjacent-level disease if symptomatic. This patient should be managed non-operatively given her absence of clinical symptoms. Serial radiographs of her whole spine should be taken to exclude atlanto-axial instability or development of scoliosis.

SUGGESTED READINGS

1. Frikha R. Klippel-Feil syndrome: a review of the literature. Clin Dysmorphol. 2020;29(1):35–7.
2. Georgiev GP, Groudeva V. Klippel-Feil syndrome with sprengel deformity. J Radiol Case Rep. 2019;13(5):24–9.

47

POST-OPERATIVE STRIDOR

You are called to urgently review a patient who earlier that day underwent a 4h anterior cervical (C3–C6) discectomy and fusion, which was reportedly completed without complications.

On examination, the patient was noted to have respiratory distress and inspiratory stridor, with a respiratory rate of 24 bpm and oxygen saturations on room air of 76%.

Q: How would you manage this patient?

This patient should be managed according to Advanced Life Support protocol using an ABC approach. I would ensure that an emergency call was put out immediately, recognising that post-operative stridor after anterior spinal surgery can progress to respiratory arrest and is a potential surgical emergency. In particular, a senior anaesthetic review would be urgently required.

Having excluded the possibility of external obstruction, for example, second to a foreign body in the mouth or upper airway, I would insert an oral airway and commence bag mask ventilation. I would ensure that appropriate cardiorespiratory monitory was commenced so I would adequately assess response to treatment.

I would continue to bag-mask the patient, monitoring saturations to ensure adequate oxygenation. Once appropriate anaesthetic support had arrived, the patient would potentially require re-intubation to protect the airway and maintain adequate ventilation. This can be performed via conventional laryngoscopy or video fluoroscopy. In an emergency after failure of intubation, in rare cases, a surgical airway can be created via a cricothyroidectomy. Emergency ventilation via this method would be performed to prevented catastrophic hypoxic brain injury because of respiratory arrest.

Following protection of the airway, I would look to identify potential surgical causes of respiratory distress. Most notably, I would want to exclude early intervertebral cage displacement, by requesting AP and lateral radiographs which could be safely performed after the patient had been intubated and haemodynamically stabilised.

Q: What are the possible causes of airway distress in a patient immediately following anterior cervical spinal surgery?

The most common reasons for immediate respiratory distress after extubation may be inadequate reversal from neuromuscular blocking agents, opioids overdose, laryngeal or bronchospasm, negative pressure pulmonary oedema and tongue fall.

However, other more specific surgical causes include local haematoma, seroma, pre-vertebral soft tissue swelling/pharyngeal oedema and implant displacement. Risk factors for this include multilevel exposure (C2–C4), prolonged surgery >5h, and blood loss >300ml.

Q: What are other potential complications of anterior cervical spinal surgery?

Causes of post-operative airway compromise following anterior cervical spine surgery occur in a predictable time sequence (Figure 47.1). Dysphagia is the most common complication. Post-operative adverse events related to the airway occur in up to 14% of patients after multilevel anterior cervical spinal surgery with or without fusion. Retropharyngeal oedema occurs in up to 6% of patients, with the greatest risk arising in multilevel surgery. A post-operative hematoma occurs in up to 2.4% in anterior cervical spinal surgery.

DOI: 10.1201/9781003201304-56

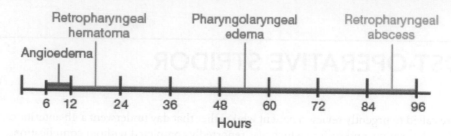

Figure 47.1 Time sequence of complications after anterior cervical spinal surgery.

Retropharyngeal abscess can be another cause of delayed airway compromise. Of patients undergoing single-level ACDF, 2% may require reintubation and as many as 5.2% may require reintubation after multilevel surgery.

A rare complication of anterior cervical spinal surgery is Horner's syndrome. This occurs due to injury to the sympathetic chain and retraction of the longus colli during the anterior approach to the cervical spine. It is thought to be most prevalent during surgery in the mid-cervical regions (C5–6).

Exam Tip

• This kind of question, while simple, has the potential to be problematic due to a lack of familiarity. Ensure that you have a working knowledge of ALS principles for this kind of scenario and go back to first principles. There can be a temptation to focus on the role you would play in a mock scenario. However, particularly for cases such as this, when other specialties would likely have the more defining role in outcomes, make sure you ask for the crash team to be called at an early stage!

SUGGESTED READINGS

1. Debkowska M, Butterworth JF, Moore JE. Acute post-operative airway complications following anterior cervical spine surgery and the role for cricothyrotomy. J Spine Surg. 2019;5(1):142–54.
2. Yee TJ, Swong K, Park P. Complications of anterior cervical spine surgery: a systematic review of the literature. J Spine Surg. 2020;6(1):302–22.

48

EPIDURAL HAEMATOMA

A 64-year-old lady presented for elective posterior cervical instrumented decompression and fixation for cervical stenosis (Figure 48.1). Pre-operatively, she complained of bilateral reduction in grip strength, weakness in shoulder abduction and ataxia. She was Hoffman's test positive with bilaterally brisk reflexes at the knee and ankle and grade 4+ power in her lower limbs.

Pre-operative blood tests, including full blood count, renal and liver profiles were normal.

There were no intraoperative complications. Estimated blood loss was 150ml, and a subfascial wound drain was inserted.

Seven hours after completion of surgery (2 a.m.), you are asked to review the patient. She has 100ml of blood in the drain. On examination, she has reduced sensation in both legs with a poorly defined dermatomal distribution and Medical Research Council (MRC) grade 1 power in hip flexion and knee flexion/extension. She has bilaterally brisk reflexes in both upper and lower limbs. She complains of worsening pain in the neck. She is apyrexial and remains haemodynamically stable.

Q: What are the differential diagnoses, and what investigations would you perform?

This patient has an acute post-operative deterioration in neurological function. The most likely diagnosis is of an epidural haematoma. Pain inhibition can lead to the false perception of weakness when testing limb movement, but this is a diagnosis of exclusion. Iatrogenic SCI should also be excluded.

I would order an urgent MRI scan of the cervical spine (Figure 48.2) to identify possible epidural collection and/or spinal cord compression.

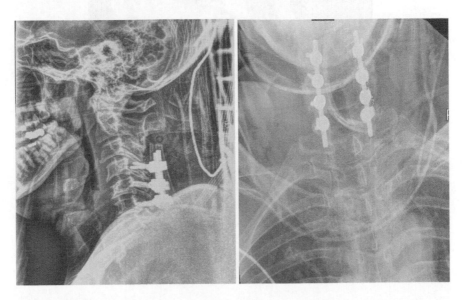

Figure 48.1 X-ray cervical spine lateral and AP after multilevel posterior decompression and instrumented fusion.

DOI: 10.1201/9781003201304-57

Q: How can neurological function be classified?

There are several separate scoring symptoms of neurological function. The Frankel grading is commonly used. According to the Frankel grading, patients are divided into five categories:

- Grade A—complete motor and sensory loss
- Grade B—some preserved sensory function with complete paralysis
- Grade C—sensory and some motor function but the motor function was of no practical use
- Grade D—sensory and useful motor function
- Grade E—normal sensory, motor and sphincter function

The American Spinal Cord Injury Association (ASIA) score is specifically for SCI and so is not designed for this patient group.

Q: What are the risk factors for the development of epidural haematoma?

The reported incidence of symptomatic postoperative epidural haematoma in the literature varies significantly from 0.1–1%. Current literature reports excess alcohol intake, age >60 years, pre-operative NSAID use, Rh-positive blood type, involvement of >5 operative levels, pre-operative Hb <10g/dL, blood loss >1L and pre-operative coagulopathy as risk factors for developing epidural haematoma.

Several studies have excluded an association between the use of post-operative drains and epidural haematoma, but there are suggestions from some studies that overuse of thrombin containing haemostatic agents may increase the risk of epidural haematoma in some cases, since early clotted haematomas are unable to drain through suction drains.

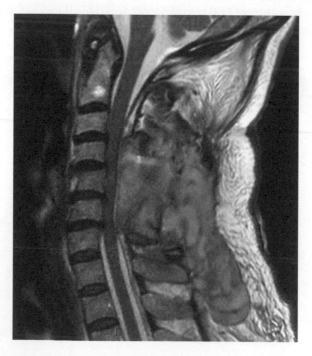

Figure 48.2 Sagittal MRI scan cervical spine (T2-weighted) showing large post-surgical collection extending into the epidural space causing spinal stenosis.

Q: What does this MRI scan show?

There is a post-surgical collection extending into the epidural space with compression of the cervical spinal cord from C4 to C6. A drain is in situ with the tip within the collection.

Q: How should this patient be managed?

Epidural haematoma causing cervical stenosis and neurological symptoms is a surgical emergency. Amiri et al. reported that patients who had their evacuation surgery within 6h of the start of their symptoms recovered a median of 1 Frankel grade more compared with those who had their surgery 6h or more after the start of their initial symptoms.

Rapid evacuation has been shown to result in better neurologic recovery by several authors. In most cases evacuation of hematoma improved patients' neurologic condition, even after a prolonged period of maximum neurologic deficit.

This patient was managed via a posterior decompression of the cervical epidural haematoma.

Exam Tips

- Spinal epidural haematoma (SEH) is a surgical emergency. SEH originates from the venous plexus of the epidural space. The most common area involved is the thoracic spine, where the epidural space is most prominent. Post-operative epidural hematomas should be suspected in the patient who either demonstrates a new post-operative neurologic deficit or develops deficits in the immediate postoperative period that are consistent with CES.
- MRI features are quite specific for haemorrhage, including isointense signal on T1-weighted images, high signal on T2-weighted images in acute cases and increased signal intensity on both T1- and T2-weighted images in subacute cases.

SUGGESTED READINGS

1. Amiri A, Fouyas I, Cro S, et al. Postoperative spinal epidural hematoma (SEH): incidence, risk factors, onset, and management. Spine J. 2013;13:134–40.
2. Ahn DK, Shin WS, Kim GW, et al. Postoperative spinal epidural hematoma: the danger caused by the misuse of thrombin-containing local hemostatics. Asian Spine J. 2017;11(6):898–902.

49

SPINAL CORD MONITORING

You are the assisting surgeon in a surgical correction of an adolescent idiopathic scoliosis.

Q: What is the role of intra-operative spinal cord monitoring (SCM) in such procedures?

SCM is used when the spinal cord is at risk for damage during a surgical procedure. Its aim is to reduce the incidence of perioperative injury to neural structures. Several established technologies are available, and combined motor evoked potentials (MEPs) and somatosensory evoked potentials (SSEPs) are considered mandatory for practical and successful SCM. Spinal cord evoked potentials are elicited compound potentials recorded over the spinal cord.

The challenge is to detect, in real time, the occurrence of neurological impairment at onset to remedy the problem as quickly as possible before it becomes irreversible.

The most common forms of SCM are

- EMG,
- SSEPs assess the functional integrity of sensory pathways from the peripheral nerve through the dorsal column and to the sensory cortex and
- MEPs consist of spinal, neurogenic and muscle MEPs. MEPs allow selective and specific assessment of the functional integrity of descending motor pathways, from the motor cortex to peripheral muscles.

Q: How does SCM work?

1. SSEPs monitor the function of dorsal column sensory pathways of the spinal cord (Figure 49.1). Signal initiation in the lower extremity usually involves stimulation of the posterior tibial nerve behind the ankle. Signal initiation in the upper extremity usually involves the stimulation of ulnar nerve. Signal recording is via transcranial recording of the somatosensory cortex.

   SSEPs are unaffected by anaesthetic or paralytic agents, but they do not monitor anterior spinal cord pathways (e.g. in cases of ischaemic injury).

2. MEPs monitor lateral and ventral corticospinal tract of the spinal cord. Signal initiation is via transcranial stimulation of the motor cortex. Muscle contraction in the extremities is measured (e.g. gastrocnemius, soleus, extensor hallucis longus of lower extremity). MEPs are more effective in monitoring the anterior spinal cord pathways (e.g. in a suspected ischaemic injury to the anterior 2/3 of the spinal cord due to infarction of the anterior spinal artery). However, MEPs are vulnerable to changes in anaesthesia.

3. EMG allows the monitoring of a specific nerve root. It can be divided into mechanical or electrical. Both forms of EMG can be overly sensitive.

   Microtrauma to the nerve root during surgery causes depolarisation and a resulting action potential in the muscle that can be recorded.

   a. Mechanical stimulation (surgical manipulation) of nerve root causes signal initiation, while the signal is recorded by muscle contraction in extremity.

   b. Electrical electromyography allows detection of a breached pedicle screw. Bone conducts electricity poorly so an electrically stimulated pedicle screw that is confined to bone will not stimulate the nerve root.

If there is a breach in a pedicle, stimulation of the screw will lead to activity of that specific nerve root. The signal is initiated via electrical stimulation of placed pedicle screw and recorded via muscle contraction in the extremity.

During the procedure and after immediately correction of deformity, you are informed that SSEP signals 'have been lost'. What should be done at this stage?

The loss of neuromonitoring signals should be taken seriously as it can be a sign of spinal cord injury (SCI). It can be managed according to a stepwise algorithm (Figure 49.2).

Step 1: Check equipment for malfunction. Electrode dislodgement from the scalp (in the case of SSEPs) or the muscle (in the case of compound muscle action potentials) can frequently occur during surgery, especially with mechanical manipulation of the spine and positioning of the patient on the operating table.

Step 2: Assess for changes in anaesthesia. Inhaled agents are known to alter SSEP and MEP characteristics. These effects tend to be more pronounced in MEPs. Similarly, muscle relaxants tend to affect MEPs, given MEPs' reliance on compound muscle action potential generation.

Step 3: Optimise cord perfusion environment. Mean arterial pressure should be elevated to 80–90 mm Hg, any anaemia with haemoglobin below 8 mg/dL should be reversed, and patient oxygenation should be increased.

Step 4: Reverse manipulation and widen decompression. It is important to address, or if possible, reverse, the offending step. For example, if the signal change developed after compression or distraction across a spinal level, then it is important to reverse that manipulation.

Step 5: Stagnara wake-up test. First described by Vauzelle et al. in 1973, this is the "gold standard" for ultimate assessment of functional integrity of the spinal cord during surgery. It requires partially awakening the patient intraoperatively to test motor function. Although the test does not provide information on sensory pathways, it provides an assessment of motor function, indicating any potential injuries to the cord.

The use of step 5 is controversial and considered outdated by many surgeons. It is also cumbersome, cannot be performed repeatedly and does not give real-time results as substantial time may elapse between injury and deficit detection.

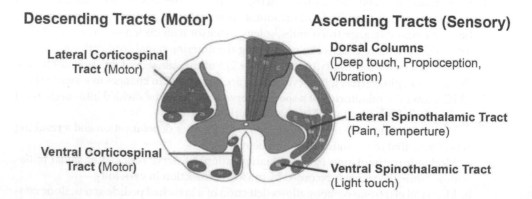

Figure 49.1 Ascending and descending tracts of the spinal cord.

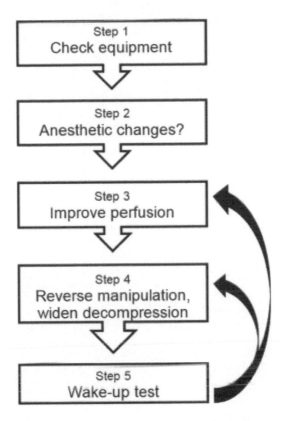

Figure 49.2   Recommended steps after loss/significant reduction of signals on spinal cord monitoring.

SUGGESTED READINGS

1.   Schwartz DM, Auerbach J, Dormans JP, et al. Neurophysiological detection of impending spinal cord injury during scoliosis surgery. J Bone Joint Surg Am. 2007;89(11):2440–9.
2.   Hilibrand AS, Schwartz DM, Sethuraman V, et al. Comparison of transcranial electric motor and somatosensory evoked potential monitoring during cervical spine surgery. J Bone Joint Surg Am. 2004;86(6):1248–53.
3.   Jain A, Khanna AJ, Hassanzadeh H. Management of intraoperative neuromonitoring signal loss. Semin Spine Surg. 2015;27(4):229–32.

50

INTERVERTEBRAL DISC ANATOMY

Q: What is the structure and function of the IV disc (Figure 50.1)?

The intervertebral disc is a heterogeneous structure that contributes to flexibility and load support in the spine. The three anatomic zones—anulus fibrosus, nucleus pulposus and cartilage endplates—are structurally and mechanically quite distinct but also highly coupled so that together they contribute to mechanical functions.

- Annulus fibrosus

The annulus fibrosus is a lamellar, fibrocartilaginous structure that is highly organised into distinct lamellas, containing large collagen fibre bundles oriented at 28–43 degrees to the transverse plane of the spine.

Its highly organised structure produces material behaviour that is anisotropic, principally in tension. It is significantly loaded in tension during physiologic motion due to swelling effects in the nucleus pulposus, as well as applied compressive loads that cause annular bulging and deformation:

- Encases the nucleus pulposus
- Composed of type I collagen that is obliquely oriented, water and proteoglycans (PGs)
- High tensile strength and able to prevent intervertebral distraction
- High collagen/low PG ratio
- Fibroblast-like cells produce type I collagen and PGs

- Nucleus pulposus

In the non-degenerate intervertebral disc, the nucleus pulposis is a shiny and gelatinous material containing a high concentration of water, negatively charged glycosaminoglycans (GAGs), collagens and non-collagenous proteins:

- Central portion of the intervertebral disc that is surrounded by the annulus fibrosis
- Composed of type II collagen
- Hydrophilic matrix (88% water) responsible for height of the intervertebral disc
- Characterised by compressibility. It is a hydrated gel due to high polysaccharide content and high water content
- PGs interact with water and resist compression. For example aggrecan is a PG primarily responsible for maintaining water content of the disc
- Viscoelastic matrix distributes the forces smoothly to the annulus and the endplates
- Low collagen/high PG ratio
- Chondrocyte-like cells survive in hypoxic conditions and are responsible for producing type II collagen and PGs

- Cartilage endplates
  - Intervertebral discs are attached to vertebral bodies by hyaline cartilage

DOI: 10.1201/9781003201304-59

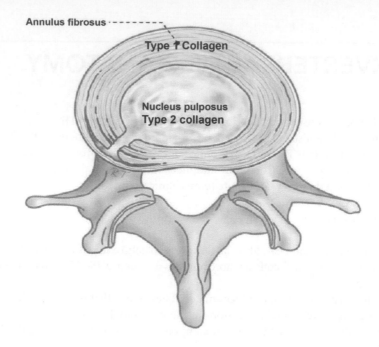

Figure 50.1   Structure of the intervertebral disc (axial view).

Q: What is the blood supply of the IV disc (IVD)?

The intervertebral disc is avascular with capillaries terminating at the endplates. Nutrition reaches the nucleus pulposus through diffusion through pores in the endplates as the annulus fibrosis is not porous enough to allow diffusion.

Q: What biological changes are seen in IVD degeneration?

Degeneration of the IVD is associated with pathologic changes in both the biochemistry and structure of the extracellular matrix. Although there is great variability in the presentation of these pathologic changes, loss of disc hydration, decreased disc height, loss of PG content, increased anulus lamellar disorganisation and decreased cell density are among the most dramatic and consistent changes.

SUGGESTED READING

Setton LA, Chen J. Cell mechanics and mechanobiology in the intervertebral disc. Spine (Phila Pa 1976). 2004;29(23):2710–23.

THINGS YOU SHOULD KNOW!

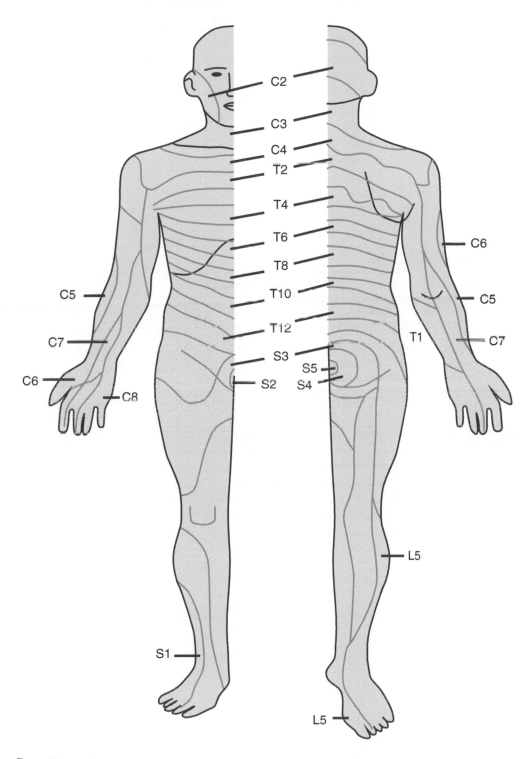

Dermatome map

Nerve Root Motor Function

Nerve Root	Motor Function
C5	Shoulder abduction
C6	Elbow flexion and wrist extension
C7	Elbow extension and wrist flexion
C8	Finger flexion
T1	Finger abduction
L1/2	Hip flexion
L3	Knee extension
L4	Ankle dorsiflexion
L5	Great toe dorsiflexion
S1	Great toe plantar flexion

Nerve Root Motor Function

Root Value	Tendon Reflexes
C5	Biceps
C6	Brachioradialis
C7	Triceps
L3/4	Quadriceps
L5/S1	Achilles Tendon

MRC Grading	Description
0	No movement
1	Flicker or trace of contraction
2	Active movement with gravity eliminated
3	Active movement against gravity
4	Active movement against gravity and resistance
5	Normal power

INDEX

Page numbers in *italics* indicate figures. Numbers in **bold** indicate tables.